Preventing
AIDS

A Sourcebook for Behavioral Interventions

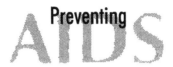

Preventing AIDS

A Sourcebook for Behavioral Interventions

Seth C. Kalichman

Center for AIDS Intervention Research (CAIR)
Medical College of Wisconsin
and
Georgia State University

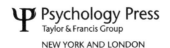

Ψ Psychology Press
Taylor & Francis Group

NEW YORK AND LONDON

First published 1998 by Lawrence Erlbaum Associates, Inc.

Published 2014 by Psychology Press
711 Third Avenue, New York, NY, 10017

and by Psychology Press
27 Church Road, Hove, East Sussex, BN3 2FA

*Psychology Press is an imprint of the Taylor & Francis Group,
an informa business*

Cover Design by Kathryn Houghtaling Lacey

Library of Congress Cataloging-in-Publication-Data

Kalichman, Seth C.
Preventing AIDS: a sourcebook for behavioral interven-
    tions / by Seth C. Kalichman.
p.   cm.
Includes bibliographical references and index.
ISBN 0-8058-2490-1 (cloth   ). — ISBN 0-8058-
    2491-X (pbk.   )
1. AIDS (Disease) — Prevention.   2. AIDS (Disease) —
    Risk factors.   I. Title.
RA644.A25K355   1998
616.97'9205—dc21   97-39257
                                                CIP
ISBN 978-0-805-82491-9 (pbk)

*Dedicated to
Hannah Fay for her inspiration
and to
the memory of Michael Morgan*

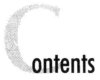

Contents

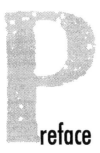reface

According to the World Health Organization, more than 10 million people have AIDS worldwide and an estimated 31 million people in the world are HIV infected (Mann & Tarantola, 1996). Since the first five cases of AIDS were described in 1981, there have been hundreds of thousands of people diagnosed with AIDS in the United States, more than half of whom have died (Center for Disease Control and Prevention [CDC], 1997). The AIDS epidemic has slowed in certain segments of the U.S. population, but there continues to be between 40,000 and 80,000 new HIV infections in the United States each year. Figure P1 illustrates the rapid accumulation of people diagnosed with AIDS in the United States, showing that the first 100,000 cases of AIDS occurred in the first decade of the epidemic and the second 100,000 cases were diagnosed shortly thereafter. Today, HIV infection is among the leading causes of death for people aged 25 to 44 years old in the United States, often exceeding deaths caused by other diseases and accidents. Thus, unlike other major causes of death that remain relatively stable from year to year, the exponential growth curve of AIDS has created a truly global public health crisis. Also setting HIV infection apart from other leading causes of death is that the causal agent is transmitted from person to person, albeit through only a few well-established modes of transmission.

AIDS was first identified in 1981 as a cluster of relatively rare infections among young men in Los Angeles who apparently shared only their sexual orientation in common; and, as it turned out, some of the same sex partners. These same mysterious diseases soon appeared in New York City and San Francisco (CDC, 1981a, 1981b). In each case, there was evidence that a badly damaged immune system afforded normally controlled infectious agents the opportunity to cause illness. AIDS had already ravaged Central Africa, and factors such as transcontinental travel, public apathy, and political indifference assured the rapid spread of AIDS across North America and most of

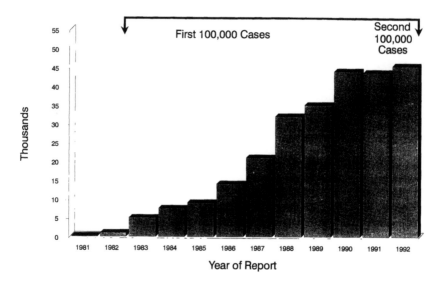

FIG P.1. Cumulative AIDS cases in the United States.

Europe. Just three years later HIV-1[1] was found to cause AIDS. The discovery of the AIDS virus led to a blood test that detected antibodies produced by the immune system that fight HIV infection. Epidemiologists showed evidence for how the virus was transmitted and, just as important, how it was not transmitted. Knowing the cause of AIDS laid the foundation for research and development of preventive vaccines, the most potent means for stopping the spread of AIDS. Despite many promising leads, however, there is still not a feasible preventive vaccine expected in the foreseeable future. HIV vaccine development has been hampered by the complexities of the virus itself, particularly the enormous genetic variation found among strains of the virus. HIV rapidly mutates, allowing new genetic subtypes to evade vaccines developed from information that can only be gleaned from preceding variants. A lack of adequate animal models for vaccine research, the ability of HIV to hide inside cells for long periods of time, and our limited knowledge of natural protective mechanisms against HIV infection present significant barriers to developing a vaccine against HIV (Essex, 1995; Working Group, 1994). Still, there has been progress, and an HIV-preventive vaccine will likely one day be a reality (Grady, 1995). Even when available, however, preventive vaccines will not offer 100% protection against HIV infection, and it is unlikely that a vaccine will be available or used by most persons at highest risk for contracting HIV. Changing HIV risk behaviors in persons at greatest risk must be kept at the forefront of efforts to prevent AIDS.

---

[1]From this point forward, HIV will refer to HIV-1 infection.

Preventing AIDS: A Sourcebook for Behavioral Interventions reviews what we know and what we do not know about the behavioral prevention of HIV infection. Recognizing that this book is a mere snapshot of the always changing landscape of AIDS prevention, I hope that new and innovative approaches to HIV risk reduction may be stimulated by examining what has been done. This book focuses on behavioral interventions aimed to reduce sexual risk. There are several reasons for selecting this focus. First, great progress has been made in stemming the transmission of HIV through blood transfusion by effectively screening the blood supply, and HIV transmission during pregnancy and childbirth has been reduced through the use of antiretroviral drugs. However, these advances will not be reviewed here because screening blood and administering antiretroviral drugs are not behavioral interventions. In addition, syringe exchange and syringe cleaning programs for injection drug users are known to effectively prevent HIV infections, but these interventions rely on changes in public policy to a greater extent than individual behavior change. Great success in preventing HIV infection through both syringe cleaning and syringe exchange has been widely documented (for a review of injection drug use and HIV prevention see Normand, Vlahov, & Moses, 1995). Reducing one's sexual risk for HIV on the other hand, is entirely dependent on individual behavior change and has been more difficult to achieve.

To guide the structure of this book, I adopted a model of innovation development processes proposed by Rogers (1995b), where interventions are diffused across social systems through a sequence of steps. In this model, a need or problem, such as risks and associated risk factors for HIV infection, is first recognized, stimulating basic and applied science in search of solutions. Research is responsible for technical advances to meet the needs and solve identified problems. In HIV prevention, research is conducted to test theories of behavior change, derive principles of behavior change, and evaluate behavior change interventions. Development of technological advances is the process of putting ideas into a form that facilitates potential use. In HIV prevention, interventions tested in controlled studies and through careful program evaluation must be recreated for specific target groups and packaged for dissemination. The diffusion and adoption of interventions requires that technology gain clearance and acceptance, for example, through reviews of scientific literature, product approval, reviews by funders, or professional consensus. Once disseminated and adopted, interventions have consequences, potentially on the targeted needs and problems. However, the consequences of HIV prevention can only be known through careful program evaluation and synthesis of available research. The innovation development process provides a useful heuristic for this book. Specifically, chapters 1 and 2 review what is known about HIV risk behaviors and factors associated with HIV risk behaviors, representing the needs and problems in HIV prevention. Basic and applied research along with development and commercialization are discussed in chapters 3 through 6, which evaluate HIV prevention intervention development and interventions designed for individuals, small groups, and communities. Finally, chapter 7 overviews the relationships among HIV prevention sciences and practices and models of HIV prevention technology transfer.

My purpose in writing *Preventing AIDS* was to provide a review of what has been done in the hope of challenging us to do what must still be done. Like the virus itself, the behavioral and social aspects of the HIV epidemic are constantly changing. Rather than discovering certain interventions that work at a given time and place, the development and dissemination of effective behavioral AIDS prevention strategies is an ongoing process. Hopefully this book will be of use in that process.

ACKNOWLEDGMENTS

I could not have completed this book without the support of many. First, I thank my research team: Charsey Cherry, Ernestine Williams, Lisa Belcher, Dena Nachimson, James Austin, and the other staff and students at the Southeast HIV-AIDS Research and Evaluation (SHARE) Project at Georgia State University for stimulating many of the ideas in this book. I am grateful for the valuable time with my colleagues Kathy Sikkema, Tony Somlai, Tim Heckman, David Rompa, and Brenda Coley at the Center for AIDS Intervention Research (CAIR), Michael Carey and Blair Johnson at Syracuse University, Roger Roffman and Joe Picciano at the University of Washington, Judith Greenberg and David Holtgrave at the CDC, Debra Murphy at UCLA, and David Ostrow at the Howard Brown Health Clinic in Chicago. I am especially indebted to Jeffrey A. Kelly for allowing me to be part of his pioneering research and for mentoring my career in AIDS. Thanks to Renee Mauroy and Moira Kalichman who helped in manuscript preparation and editing. I also thank Leslie Brogan and the Peer Counselors at the AIDS Survival Project of Atlanta for their expertise and resources. The research for this book was supported by grants R01-MH53780 and R01-MH57624 from the National Institute of Mental Health (NIMH). The Office on AIDS at the NIMH, Ellen Stover, PhD, Len Mitnick, PhD, Willo Pequegnat, PhD, and Diane Rausch, PhD, helped fuel many of my ideas by inviting me to participate in the HIV Behavioral Prevention Consortium, HIV Prevention Technology Transfer Consortium, The NIH Consensus Development Conference on Interventions to Prevent AIDS Risk Behaviors, and other meetings I have been privileged to attend. I am grateful to Judi Amsel, Kathy Dolan, Eileen Engel, and the production staff at LEA for their work in turning my manuscript into this book. I also thank Lawrence Erlbaum and Andy Baum for their support and encouragement of this project. Finally, I thank Moira, Hannah, Syd, and Rita, and the rest of my family for their endless love, support, and patience.

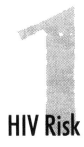

HIV Risk

HIV infection occurs when sufficient amounts of the virus are exposed to infectable cells. HIV only binds to cells carrying a specific receptor site, the CD4 molecule and associated proteins, on their surface membrane. Only a few types of cells carry CD4, including T-helper lymphocytes, monocytes, and macrophages, all of which are found circulating throughout the body as essential elements of the human immune system. The CD4 molecule is also on the surface of Langerhans cells and M-cells that are found in mucous membranes (Ayehunie, Groves, Bruzzese, Ruprecht, Kupper, & Langhoff, 1995; Soto–Ramirez, Renjifo, McLane, Marlink, & O'Hara, 1996), whose purposes are to clear potential causes of disease from mucous linings and carry them to the immune system. T-helper lymphocyte cells (T-helper cells) respond to foreign agents and direct immune reactions to neutralize potential causes of disease. HIV selectively infects and destroys T-helper cells and other cells that protect the body from viruses and other infectious agents.

Most of what is known about HIV transmission was learned from laboratory studies of transmission dynamics and through epidemiological studies examining risk histories of HIV infected people. Interviewing people who have HIV infection provides reasonable information about their behavior over the time in which they were infected. Patient interviews may also provide information about sexual partners, helping to identify sexual contacts through which HIV is spread. In addition, epidemiologists have gained considerable information from studies that simultaneously track behaviors and HIV infections as they occur in longitudinal cohorts of at-risk populations. These studies link behavior patterns and HIV transmission. Both cross-sectional and longitudinal cohort research have provided many insights into the behaviors that pose the greatest risks for sexual transmission of HIV.

Risks for HIV infection are determined by co-occurring biological factors, such as infectiousness of the HIV seropositive partner, co-occurring STDs, and integrity of genital mucosa, that facilitate HIV transmission during various behavioral practices. Exogenous psychosocial factors, such as substance use and relationship status, may also promote HIV transmission risk behaviors. In addition to biological and psychosocial factors, a third dimension that influences HIV transmission risk is the prevalence of HIV in a population; greater population prevalence of HIV increases the probability that a given sex partner in a geographic location is carrying the virus. Subpopulations with increasing incidence of HIV infection therefore suggest higher-risk for continued spread of the virus and represent priority populations for HIV prevention interventions. This chapter reviews the HIV transmission risks associated with specific behaviors, behavioral correlates, and subpopulations at greatest risk for HIV infection.

SEXUAL RISK BEHAVIORS

Any behavior that affords exposure to body fluids carrying HIV could, theoretically, result in HIV transmission. However, because a sufficient amount of virus must be present for HIV infection to actually occur, although the exact dose is unknown, only three body fluids are sufficiently concentrated with HIV to cause significant risk for sexual transmission of the virus: blood, semen, and vaginal fluids. In contrast, saliva, urine, and feces in the absence of blood do not contain sufficient concentrations of HIV to allow HIV transmission. A significant amount of attention has been given to the study of potential risks posed by saliva because frequent acts such as kissing and oral–genital contact, as well as casual contacts, can involve excessive amounts of saliva. But without the presence of blood, saliva itself does not have significant concentrations of HIV to cause risk for HIV transmission. Saliva also contains enzymes that inactivate the virus, further decreasing risks for HIV transmission (Bergey, Cho, Hammarskiold, Rekosh, Levine, Blumberg, 1993). Therefore, only sexual behaviors that allow HIV infected blood, semen, or vaginal fluids adequate access to infectable cells (those carrying CD4 on their surface membranes) should be considered HIV risk behaviors: specifically anal intercourse, vaginal intercourse, and oral–genital contact.

Anal Intercourse

Epidemiological researchers knew sex among homosexual men was the means by which AIDS was spreading well before HIV itself was discovered. The common denominator linking the first cases of AIDS was the sexual connections among its victims; infected men who engaged in anal intercourse with other men. Anal intercourse results in the deposit of semen in the rectum as well as exposure of the penis to rectal mucous linings and blood, bringing infected fluids in close contact with infectable cells (Caceres & van Griensven, 1994; Darrow, O'Malley, Byers, Echenberg, Jaffe, & Curran, 1987; Winkelstein, Samuel, & Podian, 1987). The connection between anal sex and HIV transmission is so close that as rates of receptive anal intercourse decline in populations, there is a corresponding reduction in HIV infections (Fordyce, Williams, Surick, Shum, Quintyne, 1995).

Risks associated with anal intercourse result from sufficient concentrations of HIV in semen and blood being introduced into the highly vascularized anal cavity, allowing for HIV absorption into the blood stream. Although risks posed to insertive partners during anal intercourse may be considerably lower than risks to receptive partners (Caceres & van Griensven, 1994; Ostrow, Di-Franceisco, Chmeil, Wagstaff, & Wesch, 1995), insertive partners are also at high risk for HIV infection. Risks posed to insertive partners during anal intercourse result from exposing HIV-infected rectal blood to the penile mucous membranes that contain CD4-carrying Langerhans cells. Transmission may also occur through microlacerations on the outer surface of the penis, a common occurrence during anal intercourse. Insertive anal intercourse carries risks for HIV infection independent of receptive intercourse (Coates, Stall, Kegeles, Lo, Morin, 1988; Kingsley, Detels, Kaslow, Polk, Rinaldo, 1987; Samuel, Hessol, Shiboski, Eagel, Speed, & Winkelstein, 1993). In fact, there has not been a single epidemiological study that contradicts the risks for HIV infection posed by anal intercourse.

Longitudinal cohort studies have supplied the greatest amount of evidence for HIV transmission efficiency of anal intercourse. Among 87 young men followed in a New York City cohort, Dean and Meyer (1995) found anal intercourse the most likely source of HIV transmission and reported a resurgence in rates of anal intercourse in the early 1990s. Similarly, Ostrow et al. (1995) reported that receptive anal intercourse with multiple sex partners was the best predictor of HIV infection among 68 men who became infected while under observation in a Chicago cohort. Although anal intercourse is practiced with greater frequency among homosexual men than heterosexuals, anal intercourse carries equivalent risk for HIV transmission in male–female dyads. Both men and women who engage in anal intercourse with an HIV infected sex partner are at considerable risk for HIV infection (Nicolosi, Musicco, Saracco, & Lazzarin, 1994).

Vaginal Intercourse

HIV transmission during vaginal intercourse was evident very early in the AIDS epidemic, particularly among male injection drug users and their sex partners. The heterosexual AIDS epidemic in the United States soon became apparent, and vaginal intercourse is now recognized as the principal cause of HIV infection in the world (Mann & Tarantola, 1996). Heterosexual sex accounts for 70% of AIDS cases in the world and a growing number of AIDS cases in the United States.

Risks for vaginal intercourse transmission of HIV result from similar factors as those observed in anal intercourse. Exposing either infected vaginal secretions or semen to genital mucous membranes that contain Langerhans cells, as well as microlacerations in the vaginal walls or penile tissues, allow significant concentrations of HIV to have contact with infectable cells. Laboratory studies show that vaginal mucosa absorbs simian immunodeficiency virus (SIV) in nonhuman primates (Miller, Marthas, Torten, Alexander, Moore, Doncel, & Hendricks, 1994). Vaginal HIV transmission has also been observed in artificial insemination using semen donated before HIV screening was available (Chiasson, Stonebruner, & Joseph, 1990). However, vaginal intercourse is less efficient for HIV transmission than anal intercourse because of the considerably lower likelihood of coital–vaginal bleeding in comparison to coital–rectal bleeding.

Several carefully conducted epidemiological studies have reported vaginal intercourse transmission of HIV. Research conducted with male hemophiliacs, of whom an estimated 30% to 90% were infected with HIV in the early 1980s through contaminated blood products (Chorba, Holman, & Evatt, 1993), finds significant numbers of HIV infections among their female sex partners. Studies have found as many as 10% of sex partners of HIV–infected men with blood clotting disorders are infected with HIV. More than 100 AIDS cases were reported between 1981 and 1982 in people whose only identifiable risk factor was being the heterosexual partner of an HIV infected hemophiliac (Chorba, Rickman, & Catania, 1993). Similar rates of HIV infection have been observed in heterosexual couples where one partner was infected through blood transfusion (O'Brien, Busch, Donegan, Ward, & Wong, 1994) or through injection drug use (Chiasson, Moss, Onishi, Osmond, & Carlson, 1987).

As seen with anal intercourse, risks for HIV infection are posed to both partners in vaginal intercourse. Nicolosi et al. (1994) followed couples in which the woman was HIV infected and found that 6% of their male sex partners became infected. Although other studies have reported bidirectional vaginal transmission of HIV (O'Brien et al., 1994), risk of vaginal HIV transmission is higher for the female partner. Downs and De Vincenzi (1996) found female partners in heterosexual relationships with an infected partner were more likely to be infected than male partners. Padian, Shiboski, and Jewell (1991) also reported that 20% of female sex partners of HIV-infected men contracted HIV whereas only one case of female-to-male transmission occurred. It is therefore estimated that HIV transmission is between two to four times more likely from male-to-female partners during vaginal intercourse compared to the female-to-male direction (Haverkos & Battjes, 1992). However, differences in risks should not be interpreted as men being at low risk for HIV infection during vaginal intercourse with an infected female partner; rather, men are at relatively lower risk.

Oral–Genital Contact

Despite the fact that oral–genital HIV transmission is biologically plausible when HIV infected semen or vaginal fluids are exposed to oral mucosa (Baba, Trichel, An, Liska, & Martin, 1996), early epidemiological studies failed to find associations between oral sex and HIV infection (Detels, English, Vischer, 1989; Kingsley et al., 1987; Lyman, Winkelstein, Ascher, & Levy, 1986; Schechter, Boyko, Douglas, & The Vancouver Lymphodenopathy-AIDS Study, 1985; Winkelstein et al., 1987). Laboratory research supported the low-probability of HIV transmission during oral sex by identifying only small amounts of the virus in saliva (Glasner & Kaslow, 1990; Levy, 1992), as well as identifying enzymes in saliva that inactivate the HIV (Bergey et al., 1994; Fox, Wolff, Yeh, Atkinson, & Baum, 1989; Fultz, 1986; McNeely, Dealy, Dripps, Orenstein, & Eisenberg, 1995). Later studies of couples where one partner was HIV infected and the couple only engaged in oral sex without condoms further failed to substantiate risks for HIV infection posed by oral sex (De Vincenzi et al., 1994). Additional cohort studies have reported similar findings (e.g., Ostrow et al., 1995), suggesting that risks of HIV infection through oral sex must be considered minimal.

The risk of oral–genital contact, particularly oral–penile intercourse, however, remains controversial for HIV transmission. Exposure of semen to the oral cavity has been reported as the sole risk behavior in a relatively small number of cases of HIV infection. Lifson et al., (1990) described two men who indicated semen in their mouth as their only possible risk for HIV infection over a 5-year observation period. Samuel et al. (1993) reported an additional four men who became HIV infected from the same cohort as Lifson et al. who also engaged in receptive oral intercourse and had no history of engaging in unprotected anal intercourse. Keet, van Lent, Sandfort, Coutinho, and van Griensven (1992) identified four cases, and Edwards and White (1995) reported one case of orally contracted HIV infection. Another epidemiological study has reported 4 cases of persons who seroconverted while under observation in a longitudinal cohort (Schacker, Collier, Hughes, Shea, & Corey, 1996). These case reports have led to considerable debate over the potential risks for HIV transmission posed by oral–penile intercourse.

Actual occurrences of HIV transmission during oral sex may be obscured by anal or vaginal intercourse. When oral sex occurs in the same sexual encounter as anal and vaginal intercourse, the higher-risk activities are attributed as the cause of infection. Estimating the risk of oral sex is also complicated by social pressures to deny engaging in anal intercourse because of the potential blame placed on people who practice high-risk sexual behaviors. Thus, a small number of people who admit engaging in oral sex and deny anal or vaginal intercourse may not provide accurate information about their risk histories (Brody, 1995a, 1995b). Another problem with case reports is that they do not provide information necessary for determining proportions of persons infected through oral–genital contact because the proper denominator is not known. It is therefore impossible to know the actual risks of HIV transmission through oral–penile contact.

The ambiguities of assessing risks for HIV transmission posed by oral–penile sex have led to confusion in many HIV prevention arenas. Researchers have expressed concerns about emphasizing cessation of oral sex in prevention messages, suggesting that it could be counter-productive and possibly lead to a backlash of disregard for taking any protective actions (Caceres & van Griensven, 1994). The Gay and Lesbian Medical Association (GLMA, GLMA, 1996) and the Gay Mens Health Crisis (GMHC, Nimmons & Meyer, 1996) in New York have both released position statements declaring oral sex safer and potentially safe relative to the safest of sexual practices.

Some gay advocacy groups have echoed these concerns, recommending removing oral sex from the list of risky sexual behaviors. This is an example of such sentiments expressed in an article published in the gay press:

> The Gay and Lesbian Medical Association on March 19 declared that unprotected male–male oral sex should now be classified as a "low-risk" activity for HIV transmission. Although a few documented cases of HIV transmission through oral sex have been reported, most studies have not found a statistically identifiable risk, the doctors concluded. Thus, prevention efforts should focus explicitly on unprotected anal intercourse. Benjamin Schatz, executive director of the association, said, "we believe there is a public health imperative to advocate this approach for the overall health of sexually active gay men. The confusion and mixed messages surrounding oral sex are harming our efforts to encourage gay men to make rational choices about truly risky behavior." Schatz said he hopes that prevention programs that currently characterize male-male oral sex as "high risk" or "somewhat risky" will revise their materials accordingly. Not ejaculating in the mouth further reduces the risk of HIV, the doctors said (Southern Voice, p. 12)

Only 2 months after this column was printed, a study was published in *Science* that reported oral transmission of SIV across intact oral mucous membrane in macaques, suggesting that oral transmission of HIV may rival the efficiency of rectal transmission (Baba et al., 1996). The gay press indicated there was a resurgence of fears about the risks of oral sex in gay communities.

> "The safety of oral sex has been the biggest bone of contention among AIDS educators for as long as I can remember," says Jeff Graham of the AIDS Survival Project, Atlanta. "The honest answer is that we simply do not know. I think it is ludicrous that we're so many years into this epidemic and we still don't have an answer. ... It's exactly this type of contradictory information that sends mixed messages to an already fearful public about HIV risk factors currently accepted in the medical community." (Newton, 1996, p. 9).

The tensions of how best to characterize the potential risks for HIV transmission posed by oral sex are also illustrated by the authors of a longitudinal cohort study that failed to identify evidence for oral sexual transmission of HIV and yet concluded that receptive oral intercourse should be considered a safer but not safe sexual behavior (Ostrow et al., 1995). This conclusion was again based on the biological plausibility for HIV transmission during oral–genital contact rather than epidemiological evidence for risks posed by oral sex behaviors. But despite its biological plausibility, perceptions of low risks of oral sex appear to have resulted in increased rates of unprotected oral intercourse in New York City (Dean & Meyer, 1995) and San Francisco (Schwarcz et al., 1995). A study of gay and bisexual men surveyed at a large gay pride festival in Atlanta only 2 weeks after the SIV study was published in *Science* found that 32% of men felt anxious over the potential risks of oral sex and oral–sex–anxious men were significantly more likely to report using condoms during oral sex than nonanxious men, although there were no differences in the practice of anal intercourse or unprotected oral intercourse (Kalichman, Cherry, Williams, Abush-Kirsch, & Nachimson,

1997). Thus, the unresolved issues surrounding oral sex in terms of risks for HIV infection have resulted in inconsistencies across prevention interventions regarding whether oral intercourse is treated as a high, moderate, or low risk activity. It has been common for prevention messages to convey mixed advice as to whether oral sex should be considered risky or safe.

In terms of oral–vaginal contact, there is no epidemiological evidence that suggests HIV transmission through this activity. Although also biologically plausible, women who exclusively engage in sexual acts with other women have not been found at risk for HIV infection (Cohen, Marmor, Wolfe, & Ribble, 1993; Kennedy, Scarletti, Duerr, &, 1992). For example, a study of 960,000 female U.S. blood donors did not find a single case of HIV infection among women having exclusive sexual contact with other women (Petersen, Doll, White, & Chu, and the HIV Blood Donor Study Group, 1992). These findings are supported by a study of over 1,000 women with HIV infection that found that only one woman reported sexual contact with women as her sole risk factor (Chu, Conti, Schable, & Diaz, 1994). Oral–vaginal contact, therefore appears to carry even lower risks than oral–penile contact which itself is apparently a low-risk activity.

Other Sexual Behaviors

Studies have not yet confirmed any risks for HIV transmission posed by digital–anal penetration, digital–vaginal penetration, sharing sex toys, or other such sex acts. It should be noted, however, that penetration of the anus or vagina with fingers or objects can cause trauma that is associated with increased efficiency of viral transmission during intercourse. Although women who have sex only with women may be at low risk for HIV infection, bisexual women may be at significant risk when their male partners are bisexual men or men who inject drugs. Bevier, Chiasson, Heffernan, and Castro (1995) reported that bisexual women attending a sexually transmitted disease clinic in New York City were more likely to have injected drugs, used crack cocaine, and traded sex for drugs or money than were heterosexual women attending the clinic. Seventeen percent of the bisexual women were HIV infected compared to 11% of heterosexual women.

It is also important to note that sexual risks for HIV transmission do not occur at a constant rate. Risks vary from partner to partner and from sex act to sex act with a particular partner (De Vincenzi, 1994; Joseph, Adib, Koopman, & Ostrow, 1990; Padian, Marquis, Francis, Anderson, & Rutherford, 1987; Vermund, 1996). There is also a great deal of overlap among risk behaviors, particularly injection drug use, anal intercourse, and vaginal intercourse. It is important to recognize that because people often do not become aware they are HIV infected until late in the disease process, patterns of risk for transmitting the virus to others change over time (Diaz, Chu, Conti, Sorvillo, & Checko, 1994). The prevalence of HIV in a given population and patterns of sexual mixing also change and must be considered when estimating relative risks over time. Numerous other correlates of HIV transmission result in great variability for sexual risks for HIV transmission and these factors themselves change over the course of the epidemic.

CORRELATES OF RISK

Several factors influence sexual risks for HIV transmission either by increasing the efficiency of viral transmission or facilitating risk-taking behaviors. Biological, psychological, and social correlates of HIV risk therefore create the context in which HIV transmission occurs. Figure 1.1 summarizes the array of HIV risk-related correlates. Biological and psychosocial risk factors are interactive both in and between the two respective classes. Note that I have referred to correlates rather than determinants of risk because the empirical studies that identify factors associated with risk behaviors are correlational and do not provide sufficient data to infer causal pathways. Nevertheless, consideration of these factors is essential when planning targeted HIV prevention activities.

Biological Correlates

HIV transmission is facilitated by increased concentrations of HIV in blood, semen, or vaginal fluids or by factors that increase access of HIV to infectable cells. Natural history studies of HIV infection show that the amount of HIV circulating in peripheral blood (viremia or viral load) varies over the phases of HIV infection. Higher concentrations of HIV are found in blood and semen during the first few months and at the later phases of infection. Compared to the long middle phase of HIV infection, studies have shown that men are more likely to become HIV infected when their female sex partners have advanced HIV disease (Nicolosi et al., 1994), and that the risk of women becoming infected increases threefold when their male partner has advanced HIV

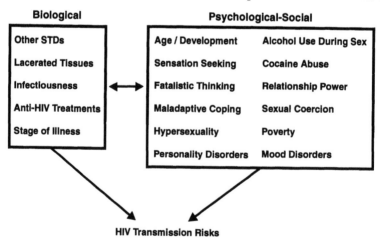

FIG. 1.1. Biological and psychosocial correlates of HIV transmission risks.

infection (De Vincenzi, 1994; Saracco, Musicco, Nicilosi, Angarano, & Arici, 1993). Sexual partners are at 6 to 17 times greater risk for acquiring HIV infection when their partner has a CD4 count below 200 cells/cubic millimeter (Royce, Sena, Cates, & Cohen, 1997).

Viral load is also affected by the person's antiretroviral medication history. Because of their inhibitory effects on the viral replication cycle, reverse transcriptase inhibitors such as AZT and D4T may reduce infectiousness of persons under treatment by lowering concentrations of HIV in blood and semen. Combination therapies that include reverse transcriptase inhibitors and protease inhibitors reduce viral load to extremely low levels, potentially offering even greater reductions in infectivity (Seage, Mayer, & Horsburgh, 1993). However, the degree to which declines in viral load are stable and offer protection against HIV transmission are not known.

Another factor affecting HIV transmission is the genetic character of the virus itself. There are numerous different genetic subtypes of HIV-1, in which there are several viral strains. There are also a number of unclassified subtypes and a group of subtypes that are outliers in terms of their genetic character, referred to as group O (UNAIDS, 1997). Subtypes of HIV vary in their binding properties, transmissibility, geographical distributions, and the manner in which they cause disease. For example, HIV-1 Subtype B is most common in the United States where sexual transmission of HIV has occurred primarily through homosexual male sex. Subtype E, however, has a strong affinity for Langerhans cells and is common in Thailand, where heterosexual transmission accounts for the majority of HIV infections (Royce et al., 1997).

HIV transmission is also influenced by the degree to which the virus can access infectable cells. Although HIV infection occurs through viral absorption by intact mucous membranes (Schoub, 1993), transmission is facilitated when mucous membranes and other barrier tissues are breached. Factors such as coital bleeding, microlacerations, tears in mucous linings, amount of coital lubrication, and even deficiencies in Vitamin A can degrade the integrity of mucous membranes and therefore enhance the efficiency by which HIV gains access to susceptible cells (Vermund, 1996). Traumatic injuries to anal and genital tissues are known to increase risks for HIV transmission. Kingsley et al. (1987) and Detels et al. (1989), for example, both showed that rectal trauma significantly increases risk for HIV transmission during anal intercourse. Similarly, vaginal bleeding during intercourse increases risks for HIV transmission (Padian, 1990). Finally, men who have uncircumcised penises may be at higher risk for contracting and transmitting HIV because of concentrations of Langerhans cells in foreskin tissue (Seed, Allen, Mertens, Hudes, & Serufilira, 1995; Urassa, Todd, Boerma, Hayes, & Isingo, 1997). Some studies estimate that HIV infection is between 1.7 and 8.2 times more prevalent in uncircumcised men compared to men who have been circumcised (Royce et al., 1997). However, the association between circumcision and HIV infection has not been consistent in the epidemiological literature (Laumann, Masi, & Zuckerman, 1997).

STDs degrade the integrity of mucous membranes and create ulcers in the genital mucosa and skin, facilitating HIV transmission (Aral, 1993). A history of STDs is a strong independent predictor of HIV infection, particularly when non-HIV infections involve genital sores, as is the case for nearly 25 million cases of genital herpes in the United States (Aral & Holmes, 1991; Aral & Wasserheit, 1995; Latif, Katzenstein, Bassett, Houston, & Emmanuel, 1989; Quinn, Glaser, Cannon, Matuszak, & Dunning, 1988; Schoenbaum, Weber, Vermund, & Gayle, 1990). Chlamydia and gonorrhea infections also facilitate HIV transmission by causing microscopic lesions in inflamed mucous membranes (Aral & Holmes, 1991). Nonulcer causing diseases form a discharge that contains infected cells or cells that are susceptible to infection. Genital ulcers further facilitate viral transmission because they provide an entry point for HIV infection and because they are likely to contain large amounts of HIV infected (or infectable) immune cells (Levy, 1992). Studies show that risk for HIV infection increases between three to five times in the presence of STDs and increased risk is greater for women than for men (Aral & Wasserheit, 1995).

Research conducted in Tanzania suggests that aggressive treatment for STDs can reduce rates of HIV transmission (Grosskurth, Mosha, Todd, Mwjarubi, & Klokke, 1995). Treatment for STDs was promoted and an intensive case management system was established in six rural communities. Incidence rates of HIV infection were monitored in these and six matched comparison communities. Results showed significant reductions in risk for the STD–treated communities and no significant changes in the comparison communities. Treatment and prevention of STDs can therefore have direct effects on HIV transmission.

STDs increase risks for HIV transmission among both homosexuals and heterosexuals (De Vincenzi, 1994; Schwarcz et al., 1995). Torian et al., (1996) found that gonorrhea and ulcerative STDs such as herpes simplex, syphilis, and chancroid disease were associated with HIV transmission risks in gay and bisexual men in New York City. Similarly, a case control study with men and women found that gonorrhea, syphilis, herpes, and genital warts were independently associated with HIV infection (Beck et al., 1996). In addition to the increased risks posed by having an infection of the reproductive tract, STDs serve as markers for unprotected sexual behaviors known to transmit HIV (Weir, Feldblum, Roddy, & Zekeng, 1994).

Psychological Correlates

Sexual risk behaviors relevant to HIV risk are known to correlate with several individual difference variables. Beliefs about AIDS, risk perceptions, and sexual motives are consistently linked to HIV risk behaviors across diverse populations. People who do not perceive themselves at risk for HIV infection or who view AIDS as a relatively minor or remote problem in the context of other issues in their lives are unlikely to take steps to reduce their risks. Studies have demonstrated that individual differences such as age, personality dispositions, psychological distress, and substance use are linked to behaviors that increase risks for HIV infection.

Age and Development. AIDS is an epidemic of the young. Forty-two percent of people with AIDS were under the age of 35 years when they were first diagnosed with an AIDS-related condition, and a full 80% were diagnosed under age 44 years (CDC, 1995a). Because it has historically taken an average of 10 years for HIV infection to cause AIDS, it is clear that most people are infected in their late teens to middle to late 20s. For this reason, sexually active adolescents and young adults in areas with high prevalence rates of infection are at considerable risk for HIV.

Studies of men who have sex with men have reliably shown that men who engage in unprotected anal intercourse tend to be younger than men who report engaging in safer sex. Age is significantly correlated with sexual risk behavior in large survey studies of men who patronize gay bars (Kelly, Murphy, Roffman, Solomon, & Winett, 1992; Steiner, Lemke, & Roffman, 1994), and one third of younger men in a San Francisco cohort were at particularly high risk for HIV infection (Lemp, Hirozawa, Girertz, Nieri, & Anderson 1994). Although studies outside the United States do not always find age associated with HIV risk in gay and bisexual men, younger men in Australia and The Netherlands also engage in higher risk sexual behaviors than do older men (De Wit, 1994, 1996; Gold & Skinner, 1994; Hospers & Kok, 1995). Age also predicts HIV risk in women. Heckman, Kelly, Sikkema, Cargill, Norman et al., (1995) found that younger women were more likely to have multiple sex partners in a recent period of time, whereas older women were more likely placed at risk because their male sex partners were known to have high-risk pasts, including bisexual and injection-drug-using histories. Thus, whereas younger men and women may be at higher risk due to patterns of sexual activity, older adults may face risks posed by longer risk histories of their male partners.

The presence of AIDS in the sexual lives of individuals changes with each passing generation. For gay men who were in their mid-20s during the sexual liberalization of the early 1980s, AIDS caused many lifestyle changes. Entire communities altered their sexual practices under the threat of AIDS. The earliest safer sex workshops and discussion groups focused much of their effort on grieving sexual losses brought on by the AIDS epidemic. In contrast, gay men in their mid-20s in the 1990s were barely teenagers when the AIDS crisis started, resulting in a generation that has grown up with AIDS. Issues of loss and grieving for men who gave up a lifestyle have been transformed into pessimism, fatalism, and apathy for many of those who have grown up in the AIDS epidemic.

Personality Dispositions. Personality characteristics including self-esteem, neuroticism, and antisocial character are well established correlates of sexual acting out. Unfortunately, much of the research in personality and sexuality has not been related to HIV risk per se. However, there is a growing literature on personality dispositions associated with risk-taking behaviors relevant to HIV risk-related practices. Impulsivity (Seal & Agostinelli, 1994) and sexual self-control (Exner, Meyer–Bahlburg, &

Ehrhardt, 1992), for example, predict patterns of sexual behavior that correspond to risks for HIV infection in relevant populations.

Propensities to take risks appear to serve as catalysts for sexual risk behaviors. The most widely studied risk-taking personality disposition is sensation seeking, which has also been identified as a correlate of sexual risk for HIV infection. Zuckerman (1971, 1994) defined sensation seeking as the tendency to peruse novel, exciting, and optimal levels of stimulation and arousal. Sensation seeking is a multidimensional personality construct that includes elements of boredom susceptibility, adventurism, experience seeking, novelty seeking, and harm avoidance, each of which have been represented in studies of sexual risk behavior of relevance to HIV risk.

Research with college students (Fisher & Misovich, 1990; Temple, Leigh, & Schafer, 1993), adolescents (Newcomb & McGee, 1991), and women (Apt & Hurlbert, 1992) demonstrates a clear association between sensation seeking and high-risk sexual behaviors. Studies of men who have sex with men have also found sensation seeking to predict risky sexual practices. Australian researchers Gold and Skinner (1992) found that young men who engaged in unprotected anal intercourse with anonymous male partners frequently endorsed statements that reflect sensation seeking; one third of men who had sex with anonymous partners reported that they did so because they were bored, wanted some excitement, and wanted an emotional boost (Gold & Skinner, 1992). Research from the Coping and Change Study cohort in Chicago reported that sexual adventurism was significantly related to the repeated practice of unprotected anal intercourse over time (Ostrow, DiFrancheisco, & Kalichman, 1997). Among heterosexual men, Clift, Wilkins, and Davidson (1993) found that men attending a genito-urinary clinic who did not consistently use condoms scored consistently higher on measures of impulsiveness and adventurism than did consistent condom users. Taken together, these findings suggest a link between personality characteristics, sexual behavior, and risk for HIV and other STDs.

Research with gay and bisexual men enrolled in safer sex workshops has also found sensation seeking to predict high-risk sex (Kalichman et al., 1994). Using a scale derived from Zuckerman's (1971) *Experience Seeking Scale* as well as a scale designed specifically to tap sensation seeking in sexual contexts and sexual sensation seeking, Kalichman, Heckman, and Kelly (1996) reported a path-analysis that showed sensation seeking significantly predicted engagement in unprotected anal intercourse, even after accounting for substance use as a part of sexual encounters. This finding suggests that sensation seeking can account for a wide range of risk-taking activities, of which sexual risk behaviors are only one behavioral domain in a more general inclination for risk taking. The interpretation that sensation seeking accounts for clusters of risk-related behaviors is consistent with theoretical formulations of sensation seeking as a trait that accounts for a spectrum of behaviors, not just sexual activity (Zuckerman, 1994). It is also consistent with theoretical biological bases of sensation seeking and by research that has identified genetic variants corresponding to personality dispositions consistent with sensation seeking (Benjamin et al., 1996; Ebstein, Novick, Umansky, Priel, & Osher, 1996).

Additional evidence for an association between personality characteristics and HIV risk behaviors is provided by research on sexual adventurism, a construct conceptually related to sensation seeking. Sexual adventurism was assessed during the first 2 years of a 9-year Chicago cohort study using items that reflected poor impulse control, risk seeking, and attraction to dangerousness in relation to a variety of sexual practices. DiFrancesico, Ostrow, and Chmiel (1996) found that men who subsequently seroconverted to become HIV-antibody positive had greater sexual adventurism scores early in the study compared to nonseroconverting seronegative controls. Seventy-nine percent of men who seroconverted scored above the median on the sexual adventurism index, compared to 44% of men who did not seroconvert. Using a 75th percentile cutoff, 50% of seroconverters were adventure seekers compared to 20% of controls, representing a 3.9 times greater risk for seronversion for men at this high range of sexual adventurism. This study provides rare evidence that risk-taking personality characteristics contribute to the incidence of HIV infection.

Another individual difference variable related to sexual risk behavior is the belief about one's future. For example, Frutchey, Blankenship, Stall, and Henne (1995) reported that many gay men in San Francisco perceived themselves as lacking a future and held fatalistic views on AIDS. These findings were subsequently confirmed by a large survey conducted with gay and bisexual men attending a gay pride festival (Kalichman, Kelly, Morgan, & Rompa, 1997). Men who engaged in unprotected anal intercourse outside of sexually exclusive relationships reported fatalistic thinking, including items such as "My future seems dark to me," and "Sometimes I feel there is nothing new to look forward to," to a greater extent than men who engaged in safer sex. These results are similar to Rothspan and Read's (1996) finding that college students with positive views of the future practiced more methods of HIV risk reduction than fatalistic students. Similarly, DiIorio, Parsons, Lehr, Adame, and Carlone (1993) reported that African-American college students who had more constricted perceptions of their future were less likely to practice safer sex than more future-oriented students. Finally, Kalichman, Rompa, and Muhammad (1996) found that scores on a fatalism scale significantly predicted engaging in sexual risk behaviors in a sample of low-income, African-American men. These findings converge to suggest that fatalistic thinking may help explain the motivation of some people who engage in high-risk sexual practices.

Coping Styles.   Individual styles of coping and managing daily stressors are associated with sexual practices. People living under impoverished or life-threatening circumstances, including those common in U.S. inner cities may engage in multiple health-compromising behaviors. Of particular relevance to HIV risk are stressful situations that may influence rates of sexual and drug-using behaviors (Cohen & Williamson, 1991). Threats associated with living in the inner city include violent crime, drug abuse, and discrimination. These experiences are linked to increased frequencies of HIV-risk behaviors among low-income men and women living in U.S. urban centers

(Kalichman, Adair, Somlai, & Weir, 1996). Early in the AIDS epidemic, Joseph, Montgomery, Emmons, Kirscht, and Kessler (1987) found that gay and bisexual men who held greater perceptions of personal risk for HIV infection reported the fewest reductions in high-risk sexual practices. In another early study, McKusick, Hortsman, and Coates (1985) found that gay men reported unsafe sexual practices with multiple partners as a means of reducing tension. High-risk sexual practices can function as coping responses in a similar manner as smoking, overeating, and substance abuse (Folkman, Chesney, Pollack, & Phillips, 1992). Living under the stress of poverty and being surrounded by high rates of AIDS can strain coping capabilities and lead to escape behaviors as a means of coping. Alcohol and other drug use can serve as a means of escaping from stressors, and substance use may increase risks for HIV infection. Therefore, limited coping capacities commonly experienced by people at risk for HIV infection impede one's ability to deal with sexually risky situations (Hobfoll, 1989; Hobfoll, Jackson, Lavin, Britton, & Shepherd, 1993).

Another way in which coping can influence HIV risk behavior is the degree to which individuals deny their personal risks for infection. AIDS has a curious way of evoking hysteria and denial, and sometimes even a strange mix of the two. In spite of the accumulation of consistent epidemiological evidence for how HIV is and is not transmitted, there are some who actually deny and even refute behaviors known to transmit HIV. Brody (1995a, 1995b), for example, argued that vaginal intercourse does not pose risks for HIV transmission and that heterosexual persons with AIDS are in fact infected through anal intercourse. Brody believed that epidemiological researchers fail to adequately assess anal sex and therefore misattribute HIV infection to vaginal intercourse. When researchers have asked about anal sex, Brody claimed that people simply do not report anal intercourse and lie to produce socially desirable responses. In addition, Brody and others (e.g., Rotello, 1997) claimed that condoms do not protect against HIV transmission, and that condom promotion amounts to nothing more than an anti-sex campaign. Despite having not published his own research and failing to cite supportive empirical studies, Brody held that his views are based on scientific evidence and that those who disagree are stating only what is politically correct. Similar to those who argue that HIV is not the cause of AIDS (Duesberg, 1988, 1989), Brody has provoked considerable interest. Unfortunately, perspectives that distract attention from the realities of AIDS can fuel denial and may do far more harm than good.

Psychopathology and Psychological Disturbances.

    Psychological disturbances that encompass hypersexuality, such as manic episodes, can directly increase risk for HIV infection in their respective symptomatology. Lack of sexual impulse control may lead to aberrant sexual acting out that can include high frequencies of sexual behaviors with multiple partners. Persistent and pervasive thoughts about sex linked with strong sexual desires and urges characterizes some psychological disturbances, such as excessive sexual-erotic ideation and sexual compulsivity (Barth & Kinder, 1987; Boast & Coid, 1994; Money, 1988, 1991). Individuals who are sexually preoccupied engage in high-risk sex despite their risks for HIV infection (Quadland, 1985;

Quadland & Shattls, 1987). These same characteristics may contribute to continued behaviors that risk infecting others after one tests HIV seropositive. In a study of over 200 HIV seropositive men participating in substance abuse support groups and HIV prevention programs, Kalichman, Greenberg, and Abel (1997) reported that 26% were having unprotected sexual intercourse with multiple partners. HIV infected men who continued to engage in high-risk sex were characterized by greater sexual compulsivity when compared to men with one or no unprotected partners. Thus, although personality characteristics such as sensation seeking appear controllable, divertable, or suppressible, sexual compulsivity and related variants of uncontrolled sexual behavior create a pervasive form of sexual risk.

People with personality disorders also report higher rates of sexual risk behaviors (Kalichman, Carey, & Carey, 1996). Poor judgment, dysfunctional relationships, and self-destructive behaviors are among the factors that may influence risk for HIV in people with personality disorders. Substance abuse and mood disturbances also co-occur with personality disorders and may contribute to associated risks. Although research has not yet discerned the specific psychiatric symptomatology or diagnostic categories that correspond to elevated risk for HIV infection, there is evidence that psychiatric populations in high-AIDS-incidence urban centers as a whole are at considerable risk for HIV infection (Kalichman, Carey, & Carey, 1996).

A number of studies have found that psychological distress is associated with increased HIV risk. Depression and anxiety correlate with high-risk sexual behaviors in samples of men who have sex with men, homosexual and bisexual adolescents, and injection drug users. Other negative moods, such as anger, have also been associated with risky sexual practices. The relationship between negative mood and sexual risk behaviors parallel the connection between stress and risky sex, where sexual activity may help people meet psychological needs through anxiety reduction and increased affection and support. Depression and anxiety can also include elements of pessimism and constricted views of the future, both of which have been associated with risk behavior. However, the exact mechanisms by which psychological distress of any form influences sexual risk have not yet been determined.

Substance Abuse. Since the earliest days of the AIDS epidemic, psychoactive substance abuse is known to correlate with HIV risk. (Stall, McKusick, Wiley, Coates, & Ostrow, 1986). A critical factor in the spread of HIV in urban centers is the use of psychoactive drugs, particularly sharing injection drug equipment (Lebow et al., 1995). Noninjection drug use, especially noninjecting forms of cocaine, is also directly associated with HIV risk. As many as 80% of crack cocaine users report histories of other STDs, and 12% of crack using men in New York City and 7% in Miami are HIV seropositive. Thus, HIV infections are over two thirds more prevalent among crack users than nonusers (Eldin, Irwin, Faraques, McCoy, & Word, 1994). Similar patterns of drug use are observed among STD clinic patients, where cocaine use is associated with syphilis and other ulcer causing STDs (Zenilman, Hook, & Shepherd, 1994). Crack cocaine is relatively inexpensive and has become one of the most widely used drugs among the inner-city poor (Eldin et al., 1994), the severely mentally ill (Meyer, Cournos, & Empfield, 1993; Susser, Valencia, & Miller, 1995), and the homeless (El-Bassel & Schilling, 1991; Kelly, Heckman, & Helfrich, 1995; St. Lawrence & Brasfield, 1995).

One study that surveyed homeless men who were receiving free meals from an Atlanta mission for the homeless showed that 65% had used cocaine in the previous 3 months (Kalichman et al., 1996). Homeless men who were cocaine users reported significantly higher frequencies of unprotected sexual intercourse, a greater number of female sex partners, and lower rates of condom use than their noncocaine-using counterparts. Even after controlling for other risk factors, men who used cocaine were three times more likely to have received money or drugs in exchange for sex and were over four times more likely to have given someone money or drugs for sex. The sexual relationships of cocaine-using men were characterized as transient and were directly associated with drug use. HIV infection among low-income men and women may therefore be best understood when examined in the context of addictive drug use, particularly cocaine.

Cocaine and HIV infection are joined because of the sexual behaviors and sexual contexts directly related to the use of this drug. Cocaine creates a sense of enhanced sexual pleasure and heightened erotic intensity (Wells, Calsyn, & Saxon, 1993). This potential aphrodisiac quality of cocaine may itself motivate its use. Perhaps more importantly is the role that cocaine plays in bartering sex for drugs; sexual commerce is an integral part of the economics of cocaine. The highly addictive potential of cocaine, especially crack cocaine, its intensive and short-lived effects, and patterns of binge use correspond to high frequencies of sex acts with multiple anonymous partners reported by crack using men and women (Auerbach, Wypijewka, & Brodie, 1994; Des Jarlais, Abdul–Quader, & Minkoff, 1991; Inciardi, 1994; Nyamathi, Bennett, & Leake, 1995; Ratner, 1993). Sexual encounters occurring in exchange for cocaine are also less likely to include the use of condoms (El-Bassel & Schilling, 1991; Susser, Valencia, & Torres, 1995). Like cocaine, methamphetamine is tied to sexual relationships through its associations with enhanced sexual sensations. Similar patterns linking drug use to sex have also been observed with respect to methamphetamine.

Studies have also pointed to noninjection drugs other than cocaine and methamphetamine as correlates of HIV risk behavior. Alcohol, for example, is the most common type of drug used in conjunction with sexual risk behavior. In addition, men who have sex with men often use nitrite inhalants (poppers) in conjunction with anal intercourse. Nitrite inhalants and MDMA (Ecstasy) are both sold specifically for use in sexual encounters and have been closely linked to unprotected anal sex with occasional partners (Ostrow et al., 1993). Nitrite inhalants are associated with anal sex because of direct pharmacological effects that induce transient states of euphoria and relax smooth muscles to facilitate anal sex. Ecstasy, on the other hand, is used to increase sexual arousal and intensity of sexual pleasure. Certain drugs, particularly cocaine, poppers, and Ecstasy are closely linked to sexual behavior, leading to their conceptualization as drugs with specific sex enhancing qualities, or sex drugs.

The use of a variety of psychoactive substances, including marijuana and alcohol, are inextricably linked to sex by virtue of their perceived sexual effects and their co-occurrence in settings where both substance use and sex take place. Drug use can become associated with sexual excitement and pleasure through associations formed with characteristics of settings and sexual feelings. Drugs can also reduce sexual anxieties and act as social disinhibitors (Leigh & Stall, 1993). Substance use can, however, be spuriously related to sexual behaviors, such as when drugs are used to cope with stress in a corresponding fashion that sex is used for coping, or when substance use and sexual behavior both stem from risk-taking personality dispositions. Types of drugs and their meaning also vary across geographical locations and cultural subgroups. The link between risky sex and drug use is well established, but there are likely multiple mechanisms and pathways through which these associations emerge.

The substance abuse–risky sex connection is, for the most part driven by the psychosocial factors previously noted. However, drugs can have biological bases for increasing risks for HIV transmission. Cocaine and nitrite inhalants, for example, may increase the permeability of mucous membranes, facilitating HIV transmission. In addition, these drugs may stimulate local immune mechanisms that have transmission-enhancing effects. Therefore, drug use is among the most complicated risk covariates, with the potential for psychological, biological, and social interactions to elevate HIV transmission risks.

Social Correlates

HIV is typically transmitted in the context of close, intimate, and private relationships. Understanding HIV risk therefore requires close attention to interpersonal relationship factors, such as power, coercion, disclosure of risk histories, and the societal forces in which HIV risk behaviors are embedded.

Relationships. The meaning of condoms and safer sex is not the same across all relationships. Love, safety, and trust can contradict the need to take self-protective actions. Condoms can therefore imply a lack of trust, posing significant barriers to their use. The need to practice safer sex in relationships tends to dissipate over time, particularly as trust develops between partners. For example, Carballo–Dieguez, Remien, Dolezal, and Wagner (1997) found that desires for sexual pleasure, intimacy, love, and trust overpower concerns about HIV risk among Puerto Rican men in partnered relationships with other men. Unprotected sexual practices occurred in coupled relationships regardless of whether one of the partners was HIV seropositive.

Across heterosexual and homosexual relationships alike, condom use is less common in steady relationships than it is in casual sexual encounters (Misovich, Fisher, & Fisher, in press). Studies of commercial sex workers show that condoms are used more frequently with paid sex contacts than with stable partners. This same pattern of condom use has been reported in studies of heterosexual couples, where condoms are used more frequently in casual than steady partnerships (Temple & Leigh, 1992). Condom use clearly carries different communicative values in steady relationships, where care, trust, safety, and commitment contradict protecting each other from each other (Misovich et al., in press). Believing that a relationship has developed into a steady partnership is the reason why many couples stop using condoms. Of course, when coupled partners are both HIV seronegative and are monogamous they are in fact at no risk for HIV infection. Unfortunately, long-term monogamy is often more of an ideal than a reality.

Power.   Cultural and socioeconomic factors strongly influence sexual decision making. Power imbalances and gender scripting determine the degree of control one has in their sexual relationships. Power and control create significant barriers to self-protective behaviors among women, particularly women living in poverty (Sobo, 1993). Amaro (1995) identified four central factors that contribute to women's sexual risk for HIV infection: (1) social status of women in a given society; (2) the importance placed on relationships in defining women's sense of self-worth; (3) the men women become involved with; and (4) history of and fear of physical and sexual abuse. Women do not have significant power to change the relationships in which they are financially dependent. Power in sexual relationships therefore plays a direct role in HIV risks. Factors that contribute to risk include sexual partners history of injection drug use and past sexual activity, the use of addictive substances in conjunction with sex, and the occurrence of sexual pressure and coercion. Although these issues have been widely discussed (Amaro, 1995; Fullilove, Fullilove, Haynes, & Gross, 1990; Sobo, 1993; Wingood & DiClemente ,1992), there has been less empirical study of how those factors influence HIV risk in sexual relationships.

More than half of women living in inner-city housing developments report at least one factor that places them at high risk for HIV infection, and the most common risk factor is their sex partner's sexual history and history of injection drug use (Kalichman & Stevenson, 1997). Kalichman and Stevenson, 1997 found that one in five women deemed at high risk for HIV infection feared abandonment if they suggested using condoms, and 10% feared that they would be hit if they requested their partner to use a condom. Women who reported being at risk for HIV infection were also more likely to have been forced or coerced into unwanted sex than women at lower risk.

Coercion.   Unwanted sexual experiences are a prevalent problem in heterosexual dating relationships, with numerous studies documenting frequent acts of sexual coercion (Baier, Rosenzweig, & Whipple, 1991; Muehlenhard, Powch, Phelps, & Giusti, 1992). For example, Koss, Gidycz, and Wisniewski (1987) found that one in four college women experienced sexual pressure and 9% had been threatened or forced to engage in sexual intercourse. Sexual coercion in heterosexual relationships is related to the use of alcohol and other drugs, power differentials between partners, and nonassertive responses to coercive pressure (Muehlenhard & Linton, 1987). Recipients of unwanted sexual advances are known to suffer psychological distress for extended periods of time as a result of their being sexually coerced. For example, Gidycz and Koss (1989) reported that female victims of sexual coercion experience symptoms of clinical depression attributable to the sexual assault.

Sexual coercion is not, however, limited to heterosexual relationships. In a small study, Mezey and King (1989) found that sexual assault against men perpetrated by men often involved the use of alcohol and other drugs and that same-sex coercion frequently resulted in serious psychological distress. Parallel to heterosexual coercion, 18 of 22 men who were sexually coerced were acquainted with the offender and 20 of the assaults involved attempted or completed anal intercourse. Waterman, Dawson, and Bologna (1989) found that forced sex was prevalent among gay male college students, with 12% of their sample reporting forced sexual experiences. Men who were forced to have sex with other men also experienced nonsexual violence. In a larger study in the United Kingdom, 27% of homosexually active men reported a lifetime history of being forced to have sex against their will, with one third of these men identifying the perpetrator as someone with whom they had had consensual sexual relations. One third of gay and bisexual men participating in an HIV prevention-intervention in the mid-Western United States reported being coerced into unwanted sexual contact; 92% of the coercive acts involved unprotected anal intercourse (Kalichman & Rompa, 1995). Thus, rates of coercive sexual behaviors in gay relationships are similar to those found among heterosexuals. Like women who experience sexual coercion, men who are sexually coerced experience greater psychological distress and have lower self-esteem than noncoerced men (Kalichman & Rompa, 1995).

Risk Disclosures. The privacy of sexual relationships often translates to secrecy about past sexual lives. The fact that people are inclined not to discuss their sexual pasts is well known (Doll, Harrison, Frey, McKirnan, Bartholow et al., 1994), and many persons would rather not know the details of their sex partners' past relationships. Bisexual men, for example, often do not disclose their same sex relations to their female partners and similarly hide their heterosexual experiences from their male partners (Stokes, McKirnan, & Burzette, 1993). In a study of bisexual men seeking HIV risk reduction services, three fourths of the men with primary female sexual partners had not disclosed their bisexual activity to their female partners and 64% had not modified their sexual behavior to protect their female partners from HIV infection (Kalichman, Roffman, Picciano, & Bolan, 1997). Failure to disclose past or present risks to sex partners can be motivated by many factors including fears of abandonment, stigmas associated with bisexuality, and being labeled promiscuous.

It is also well documented that a minority of people who have HIV infection do not disclose their HIV serostatus to their sex partners. Schnell, Higgins, Wilson, Golobaum, and Cohn, (1992) reported that 11% of HIV infected men do not disclose their HIV infection to primary sex partners. In a study of mostly low-income Hispanic men, Marks, Richardson, and Maldonado (1991) found that half had not disclosed their HIV status to at least one sex partner. In a similar study of women, one in five HIV seropositive women had not disclosed to sex partners and 13% had not disclosed being HIV infected to anyone (Simoni, Mason, Marks, Ruiz, & Reed, 1995). Notifying past sex partners about testing HIV seropositive is even less common, with one study finding that only one third of HIV seropositive men had attempted to let just one past sex partner know that they were infected (Marks, Richardson, Ruiz, & Maldonado, 1992). Subsequent studies have shown that cultural values and social pressures strongly influence self-disclosure of HIV serostatus (Mason, Marks, Simoni, Ruiz, & Richardson, 1995). In fact, Mason et al. (1995) found that disclosure of HIV serostatus coincided with disclosure of homosexual or bisexual orientation, suggesting that generally supportive environments for sexual openness and acceptance facilitate disclosure of both HIV risk history and HIV antibody serostatus.

Societal Influences. Sociocultural factors influence the sexual scripts that are played out as roles in sexual relationships (Kelly & Kalichman, 1995). Still, relatively little research has investigated societal dimensions of HIV risk in relationships, including culture, values, community norms, and public policies. The dearth of information in this area is likely attributable to difficulties in operationalizing and measuring macrosocial constructs. However, research has assessed individual perceptions of socially held beliefs about HIV risk and risk reduction behaviors. Social perceptions, particularly perceived social norms, serve to promote and reinforce sexual practices including sexual risk and sexually protective behaviors. Studies show that gay and bisexual men who perceive condoms and safer sex as being more accepted by their peers are themselves more likely to practice safer sex (Kelly et al., 1992). Steiner et al. (1994) found that perceptions of peer norms for safer sex were stronger among men who did not practice unprotected anal intercourse compared to men who practiced this highest-risk behavior. Indeed, dramatic changes in risk behavior over the course of the HIV epidemic observed among gay and bisexual men in HIV epicenters are commonly attributed to changes in social norms and redefining of sexual relationships resulting in norm changes. Similar influences of social norms on sexual behaviors have not, however, been consistently observed in studies of women at-risk. Kalichman and Stevenson (1997), for example, failed to find perceived norms to predict HIV risk behavior histories. A likely explanation for the limited influence of social norms on women's risk for HIV is the fact that much of their risk is actually determined by their partner's risk history.

Another social factor that may influence HIV risk behavior is the perceived severity of HIV infection. On a societal level, beliefs about treatments for HIV and AIDS and the potential for a cure may reduce vigilance against risky behaviors. Hope offered by protease inhibitors and other anti-HIV medications can backfire on behavioral prevention efforts. The effects of widespread cultural beliefs that a cure for AIDS is around the corner are mostly unknown and will require careful monitoring as promising new treatments are discovered.

EPIDEMIOLOGY OF HIV

Although HIV infection occurs across geographic and demographic lines, several groups have been most affected by AIDS the longest. People at risk for HIV infection are defined on the basis of the two necessary conditions for HIV transmission: the frequency of behaviors that allow efficient viral transmission and the prevalence of HIV in the population. Although defining groups as being at-risk for HIV infection loses much of its meaning as the epidemic expands, attention must be paid to segments of society with the greatest prevalence of HIV infection for prevention activities to impact the epidemic.

Men Who Have Sex With Men. The AIDS crisis in the United States occurred first among homosexually active men, and the virus has spread rapidly through anal intercourse between male partners. It is therefore important to note that although high HIV seroprevalence rates occur in gay communities, men who have sex with men are only at high risk for HIV infection when they practice anal intercourse. Across a wide array of samples and research methodologies, studies show that approximately one third of men report engaging in recent unprotected anal intercourse (Kelly, St. Lawrence, & Brasfield, 1991; Lemp et al., 1994; Ostrow et al., 1995). Unprotected anal sex commonly occurs among homosexually active men who are not gay identified. There is also a common trend toward younger gay men, generally defined as under age 30, being at higher risk than relatively older men. Although there is considerable evidence that the HIV epidemic among men who have sex with men in New York City has leveled off, rates of HIV transmission in gay and bisexual men have decreased nationally since 1985 (Mann & Tarantola, 1996; Smith, Mikl, Hyde, & Morse, 1991), and the number of homosexually contracted cases of AIDS has declined since 1991. There is, however, considerable concern that some gay and bisexual men are experiencing significant lapses to unsafe sex and that many men are unable or unwilling to stop practicing unprotected anal intercourse. A resurgence of HIV infections, or second wave, may therefore be occurring among gay and bisexual men in many U.S. cities.

Injection Drug Users. High HIV prevalence rates and frequent sharing of injection equipment create an alarming situation for persons who inject drugs and their sexual partners. Although actual rates of needle-sharing practices are not known, more frequent injectors are more likely to test HIV seropositive (Williams, 1990). Needle sharing, like sexual behavior, occurs in close, intimate, and private relationships, as well as between anonymous partners (Magura, Grossman, Lipton, Siddiqi, & Shapiro, 1989). HIV transmission is therefore linked to injection drug use through multiple pathways. Injection drug users who are infected with HIV can also infect their noninjecting sexual partners (Booth, 1988; Kane, 1991). A close association also exists between injection drug use and trading sex for drugs (Normand, Vlahov, & Moses, 1995). The types of drugs used can also synergize to compound HIV risks. For example, injection drug users who smoke crack cocaine are at greater risk for contracting sexually transmitted HIV compared to those who only inject (Booth, Watters, & Chitwood, 1993).

Heterosexual Adults. Vaginal and heterosexual anal intercourse account for most of the world's HIV infections (Mann & Tarantola, 1996). Heterosexual transmission of HIV is also responsible for a significant number of new AIDS diagnoses in the United States. Across geographic regions, heterosexuals in the United States demonstrate substantial rates of HIV risk-related behaviors. In a national telephone survey, Catania, Coates, Stall, Turner, and Peterson, (1992) found that 15% to 31% of adults practiced sexual behaviors that could create risk for HIV infection, with 7% of persons reporting two or more sexual partners in the previous year. In another nationally representative sample, Ericksen and Trocki (1992) reported that 22% of people reported two to four sexual partners in the previous 5 years. Other national surveys find similar rates of risk-related sexual behaviors practiced among heterosexuals (Billy, Tranfer, Grady, & Klepinger, 1993). As the prevalence of HIV increases among heterosexuals in North America, sexual practices that allow efficient transmission of the virus will fuel the heterosexual epidemic.

Particular attention has been given to heterosexual women infected by their injection drug using and bisexual male partners (Aral & Wasserheit, 1995). Studies of HIV transmission show that vaginal and anal intercourse are more efficient routes of HIV transmission from men-to-women than from women-to-men. However, risks of heterosexual intercourse posed to men are lower but the risks are not low. Men report greater numbers of sex partners and higher rates of sexual acts than do women (Billy et al., 1993). In addition, virtually every correlate of risk is found with greater frequency among men than women, including ulcerative STDs, noninjection substance abuse, and risk-taking personality dispositions. Women, however, are more likely to seek testing for HIV because women generally access health care more so than men and because many women are screened for HIV antibodies in reproductive and prenatal health care. HIV-infected men are therefore less likely to be detected than are women. These factors combined suggest that rates of heterosexually transmitted HIV infection will remain higher among women but numbers of men who contract HIV through sex with women will also continue to rise.

Adolescents. The average length of time between the point of HIV infection and receiving an AIDS diagnosis spans several years, so most people with AIDS in their 30s were likely infected during their teens (Hein, 1990). Approximately 17,000 people between the ages of 13 to 19 were infected with HIV between 1981 and 1987 (Gayle & D'Angelo, 1991). National rates of other STDs show that U.S. youth present the highest rates of gonorrhea of any age group (Gayle & D'Angelo, 1991). The prevalence of non-HIV sexually transmitted infections and increasing rates of HIV raise many concerns about the spread of AIDS among adolescents, especially given their frequency of sexual risk behaviors. National studies show that a majority of teens engage in sexual intercourse, and one in five have had multiple lifetime sexual partners, with those having more partners being the least likely to use condoms (Tanfer, Grady, Klepinger, & Billy, 1993). The average age of first sexual intercourse is approximately 16 years, with one third of male and one fifth of female adolescents having their first intercourse experience before the age of 15 years (Billy et al., 1993). Several lines of evidence, including increased prevalence rates of STDs and unplanned pregnancies, suggest that continued high rates of HIV will be contracted during adolescence.

People Living With HIV Infection. Research suggests that as many as one third of HIV seropositive men who have sex with men engage in unprotected anal intercourse, and the rate of risky sex among seropositive men may not be any less than that observed among seronegative men (Kelly et al., 1992; Lemp et al., 1994; Schwarcz et al., 1995). One study found that 28% of HIV seropositive men attending substance abuse support groups had engaged in multiple unprotected sex acts and 34% had two or more sex partners in the previous month (CDC, 1996). High rates of unprotected sex have also been observed among HIV seropositive men enrolled in mental health and prevention intervention trials. For example, one in five men who participated in a mental health, coping, and adjustment intervention trial had engaged in unprotected anal intercourse over a 3-month time period (Kelly et al., 1992). Similarly, among HIV seropositive gay and bisexual men enrolled in a primary prevention intervention study, 76% were sexually active, 39% reported engaging in unprotected anal intercourse in the previous 3 months, and the majority were in serodiscordant relationships (Kalichman, Kelly, & Rompa, 1997). Similar rates of continued sexual risk behavior have been observed among nongay-identified men who have sex with men and hetero-sexual homeless men (Kalichman, Belcher, Cherry, Williams, Sanders, & Allers, 1997). Although awareness of one's positive HIV serostatus results in life-long behavior change for some persons, many people living with HIV infection occasionally practice unsafe sex and are in need of risk reduction interventions as well as ongoing support for maintaining safer sex practices over their increasingly longer lifetimes.

People living with HIV infection may also engage in unsafe sex practices with other HIV seropositive persons. Seroconcordant seropositive relationships obviously do not carry risk for new HIV infections. However, the threat of co-infection with other STDs and reinfection with different variants of HIV pose health risks. Despite these risks, seroconcordant seropositive couples may choose to practice unprotected sex. Among gay and bisexual men, so-called bare-back sex has been sensationalized in the popular press. For instance, a column in Poz Magazine stated:

I'd had unsafe sex before, but never intentionally. Those experiences were guilt-ridden because I worried—both during the sex and afterward—about exposing my partner to HIV. This was different. Knowing the guy was positive made it empowering, not guilt inspiring. I relaxed into my desires instead of fighting them and felt good doing so. On a purely physical level, the experience wasn't extraordinary, but emotionally everything purred so fine. (Gendin, 1997, p. 64)

The dynamics of unprotected sex in seropositive seroconcordant relationships are clearly different from those in serodiscordant and seronegative seroconcordant couples. Preventive interventions must therefore address the specific contexts in which sex occurs.

Other Groups. Subpopulations exhibiting behavior patterns that carry significant risk for HIV transmission in closed sexual networks are appropriate targets for HIV prevention. Of particular interest are subgroups whose sexual behaviors and relationships indicate that when HIV is introduced in a sexual network, the virus will rapidly spread through efficient modes of transmission. Individuals who exchange sex for money, drugs, or survival are therefore at high risk for HIV infection. Between 15 to 55% of commercial sex workers in the United States are HIV seropositive (Campbell, 1990). Incarcerated prison inmates are at elevated risk for HIV infection because of the injection drug use and homosexual activity that occurs in closed sexual networks. The fact that condoms are considered contraband in prisons does not help matters. Nearly 4 million U.S. migrant and seasonal workers are at risk because high rates of infection occur in these closed communities. Seriously mentally ill adults, homeless adults, and transient youth, as well as other socially disenfranchised and isolated groups, are also at risk for the continued spread of HIV. Thus, as the HIV epidemic expands, people at the highest risk remain those who engage in behaviors that afford efficient viral transmission in sexual and injection drug using networks with high prevalence rates of HIV infection.

CONCLUSIONS

Little about the AIDS crisis can be considered remotely positive. But the fact that HIV is only transmitted through a few very specific practices offers our greatest hope for controlling the AIDS epidemic. Individual choices and decisions to change risk-related behaviors remain the most viable means of preventing new HIV infections. Changing sexual behaviors for the long term, however, has proven difficult. Sexual behaviors are highly reinforced and occur in complex social environments that are often resistant to change. Preventing HIV infections, however, hinges on behavioral choices to circumvent transmission. Behavior change strategies that can avert HIV transmission are therefore the primary armaments for HIV risk-reduction interventions.

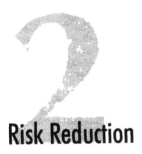

Risk Reduction

To prevent HIV transmission, one must either avoid contact with infected blood, semen, or vaginal fluids in the first place or intercept the virus after exposure but before the onset of infection. Possibilities for postexposure HIV prevention include the use of topical microbocides to prohibit HIV from binding with susceptible cells, immediate suppression of HIV via chemoprophylactic use of anti-retroviral medications, or mounting an effective immune response against the virus as achieved through a preventive vaccine. Unfortunately, technologies for postexposure prophylactics are not widely available. Behavioral interventions for HIV prevention are therefore the most viable option for reducing HIV risk.

Here I review the means by which sexually transmitted HIV infections can be prevented. Following a brief discussion of recent advances of postexposure methods, the focus shifts to behavioral methods used during sexual intercourse to lower transmission risk, including practicing nonpenetrative sexual activities that eliminate risks altogether. Increased use of condoms and nonpenetrative sex practices have been the primary targets of sexual risk-reduction interventions. Indeed, theories of behavior change adapted for HIV risk reduction invariably define their outcomes in terms of condom use, safer sex, and related practices. Behavioral change must be the bottom line for HIV prevention intervention outcomes if there is to be a true impact on the epidemic. Although changes in various correlates of risk are important in promoting behavior change, it is change in risk behavior itself that prevents infection. In addition to the behaviors that reduce HIV transmission risks, this chapter reviews the social and psychological theories that guide the development of HIV risk reduction interventions.

POSTEXPOSURE PREVENTION

When HIV is not prevented from entering the body, it is theoretically possible to prevent HIV infection by blocking its transmission, either through topical virucides or with anti-retroviral medications. Although biologically based, these two strategies have clear behavioral implications in terms of compliance, acceptance, and interactions with risk behaviors. The following sections briefly review virucidal and anti-retroviral strategies.

Virucides

As noted earlier, one means of stopping HIV transmission following exposure is to inactivate the virus before or during absorption but before HIV comes into sufficient contact with infectable cells. Because HIV's protective envelope is relatively fragile, it is vulnerable to mild detergents, suggesting the feasibility of producing preparations strong enough to inactivate the virus but not harsh enough to damage mucous membranes and other genital tissues.

Because virucides, chemicals that inactivate a virus, provide a method that allows women to exercise control over preventing HIV infection, there has been considerable effort given to developing vaginal creams and ointments to protect against mucosal transmission of HIV. In addition to microbicides that inactivate the virus, agents may be developed to interfere with absorption of HIV into mucosal tissue or to inhibit the HIV replication cycle. The spermicide nonoxynol-9 and other surfactants have virucidal properties that inactivate HIV by disrupting its viral envelope (Rosenberg, Holmes, & the World Health Organization Working Group on Virucides, 1993). The potential protection of spermicides against HIV has led to their use for additional protection against HIV transmission in combination with latex condoms. Unfortunately, there has been limited evidence that nonoxynol-9 alone is effective at preventing sexually transmitted HIV infection, and nonoxynol-9 has not increased the protection offered by latex condoms (W. Cates, personal communication, April 8, 1997). For a virucide to be effective in vivo requires complete dispersion across the vaginal or anal mucosa, including the cervix. Given the 15% user failure rates for spermicides used alone as contraceptives, virucides will have to benefit from considerable advancements in technology before they can be expected to prevent HIV transmission. Clinical investigations of vaginal microbocides have begun with very early results showing limited promise. Ideally, a safe and effective microbicide would also be colorless, odorless, nontoxic, and affordable (International Working Group on Vaginal Microbicides, 1996). In theory, a microbicide that is found effective for vaginal use may also be effective in preventing anal–rectal HIV transmission.

Anti-Retrovirals

A second postexposure strategy is the use of anti-retroviral medications to avert the onset of HIV infection. The first approved and most widely used reverse transcriptase inhibitor was zidovudine (AZT), a drug developed in the 1960s to treat nonhuman retroviruses. Numerous studies have shown that zidovudine is effective in slowing HIV progression for most people treated. Effects of zidovudine treatment include increased numbers of T-helper lymphocytes, decreased HIV activity, reduced frequency and severity of opportunistic illnesses, and improved general health status. There is also evidence that AIDS is delayed by zidovudine. Zidovudine appears to extend the survival of some people with AIDS. For example, Lemp, Payne, Neal, Temelso, and Rutherford (1990) found that patients receiving zidovudine had increased survival times across subgroups of people infected through various modes of HIV transmission. The effects of AZT on infectivity, however, are unknown.

Additional nucleoside analogue reverse transcriptase inhibiting drugs are available: zalcitabine (ddC), didanosine (ddI), stavudine (d4T), and lamivudine (3TC). Each functions similarly to zidovudine, inhibiting the action of reverse transcriptase by substituting for the usual building blocks of DNA, and therefore interfering with HIV replication. The anti-retroviral actions of ddC are enhanced when taken in combination with zidovudine. Unfortunately, ddC also has toxic side effects, including peripheral neuropathy (numbness, tingling, or pain in the hands and feet), oral ulcerations, and skin rashes. Similarly, ddI presents problems with peripheral neuropathy, diarrhea, and pancreatitis (Schooley, 1992). d4T has shown promise as an anti-retroviral treatment, although it too has potential adverse effects. Non-nucleoside reverse transcriptase inhibitors are also available for treating HIV infection. Unfortunately, like AZT and related drugs, the effects of non-nucleoside reverse transcriptase inhibitors on infectivity are not known.

Protease inhibitors such as Sanquinavir mesylate, Ritanovir, and Indinavir sulfate are another class of available anti-retroviral medications. Protease inhibitors, the first of which was approved in December 1995, are for use in combination with reverse transcriptase inhibitors (Deeks, Smith, Holodniy, & Kahn, 1997). For example, the so-called AIDS cocktail or triple-combination therapy, consists of a protease inhibitor and two reverse transcriptase inhibitors such as AZT and 3TC (Cohen, 1997). Similar to reverse transcriptase inhibitors, protease inhibitors work by disrupting the HIV replication cycle. Protease is another enzyme that is essential in the replication of HIV, but rather than acting on the process of genetic transcription, protease is necessary for breaking down viral proteins into the proper components for the maturation of new virus particles (Ho, 1996). Without protease, the structural formation and organization of viral proteins is not complete, rendering immature virus particles that are not infectious. Therefore, complementing the actions of reverse transcriptase inhibitors that have their effects in the early stages of HIV replication, protease inhibitors interrupt processes in the final stages of maturation of new virus particles. The promising combination of both reverse transcriptase inhibitors and protease inhibitors comes from delivering a double punch, hitting HIV both early and late in its replication cycle (Lipsky, 1996).

The necessity of using combinations of anti-retroviral medications to combat HIV is driven by the diversity of HIV itself. HIV rapidly replicates and adapts well to pressures posed by treatments. Over the course of 10 years, the average duration of an individual's HIV infection, the virus replicates itself thousands of times, resulting in the production of as many as 10 trillion virus particles (Ho, 1995). The reverse transcription of genetic material, specifically forming DNA from viral RNA, is prone to error. In addition to viral mutations that occur in the typical replication cycle of HIV, mutations also occur in response to specific anti-retroviral treatments. It has long been known that the use of any single drug in treating HIV infection will be of limited success, and there has been an abundance of evidence to support the use of combinations of anti-retrovirals for treating HIV (Hammer et al., 1996). The use of drugs that target HIV at different stages of its replication cycle, particularly early and late in the course of HIV infection, further decreases the ability of HIV to develop drug resistance (Cooper, 1994; Ho, 1995, 1996; Kuritzkes, 1996).

Results from clinical trials of the new combination therapies are encouraging and have revolutionized the treatment of HIV. Assisted by advances in newly developed methods for monitoring viral load (Katzenstein, Hammer, Hughes, Gundacker, & Jackson, 1996), clinical trials of combination treatments showed dramatic declines in the amount of HIV present in blood. Within 2 weeks of initiating treatment, patients showed 100-fold reduction in the amount of HIV in their bloodstream (Ho, 1996), with HIV becoming undetectable in some cases (Markowitz, Saag, Powderly, Hurley, & Hsu, 1995). There is also evidence that protease inhibitors reduce viral load in lymphatic tissue and possibly semen and vaginal secretions. However, an undetectable viral load does not mean the virus has been cleared from the body. Lower-bound thresholds for plasma RNA levels range below 500 copies/ml. In addition, viral load fluctuates and the conditions of increases and decreases in various tissues and fluids are unknown. Combination therapies may therefore reduce infectivity, but the degree to which HIV transmission risks are reduced and the factors that influence these reductions are unknown.

Research has shown that the use of anti-retrovirals such as AZT following occupational exposure to HIV, particularly needle-stick injuries, may prevent HIV infection. One study showed that administration of AZT after needle-stick injury exposure to HIV reduced transmission risks by nearly 80% (CDC, 1995b). Another example of postexposure use of anti-retrovirals is administering AZT to prevent perinatal HIV transmission. Thus, the idea behind postexposure prophylaxis (PEP) is to hit HIV hard during a window of opportunity between exposure and onset of infection (Katz & Gerberding, 1997). The use of anti-retrovirals for chemoprophylaxis in these settings has led to a call for PEP following sexual transmission risks. The potential for a so-called morning-after-pill for HIV prevention (although the course of chemoprophylaxis takes weeks) drew considerable attention when combination therapies were shown to reduce amounts of HIV to undetectable levels in blood, lymphatic tissue, and other body fluids with typically high concentrations of the virus. For example, Don Howard of ACT UP Golden Gate in San Francisco launched an initiative to bring PEP to the forefront of HIV prevention. In an editorial published in several gay newspapers, Howard (1997) wrote:

> Although there are many research questions that need to be answered, the data indicate that we may be able to stop some infections from occurring if drugs

are available within hours of exposure. And some private doctors, suspecting this to be true, are prescribing these drugs to patients who come in after a high-risk sexual exposure. (p. 10)

There are, however, several concerns about using anti-retrovirals for post-sexual exposure risks. The belief that administering drugs after sex can prevent HIV infection may lead to complacency about AIDS and counterefforts to support safer sex. Resistance and cross-resistance of HIV following such use has significant implications for the long-term benefits of anti-retroviral treatments. These and other issues caution against a rush to use effective treatments for HIV as a means of preventing infection following potential exposure.

Surveys of gay and bisexual men in large urban centers have shown that PEP is in high demand and that the men most likely to seek PEP will be those at greatest risk. For example, Kalichman (1997) reported that 3% of men surveyed at an annual Gay Pride festival had used PEP and 26% of men were planning to use PEP to try to prevent HIV infection. Compared to the 74% of men who did not plan to use PEP, those planning to use PEP were younger, less educated, more likely to use marijuana, nitrite inhalants, and cocaine in the past 6 months and were more likely to have a history of injection drug use. In addition, men intending to use PEP were also more likely to have practiced unprotected anal and oral intercourse as the receptive partner and were more likely to have multiple anal intercourse partners with whom they were receptive. Men most in need of AIDS prevention interventions were therefore the most likely to seek PEP. However, these same persons may be at greatest risk for noncompliance with the demands of PEP protocols, introducing problems of repeat requests for PEP and the potential for viral resistance to anti-HIV drugs. These findings were consistent with a study of 54 men who have sex with men in San Francisco. Dilley, Woods, and McFarland (1997) reported that advances in anti-HIV therapies are having dramatic effects on perceptions of AIDS and an increased willingness to engage in risky sexual practices. Unfortunately, the efficacy of PEP for sexual exposure to HIV is not known, but will likely be far less promising than PEP for occupational exposures.

BARRIER METHODS

Condoms became the obvious means of thwarting HIV transmission immediately on recognizing that AIDS was caused by a sexually transmitted pathogen. Condoms, particularly those made of latex, were well known to prevent sexually transmitted bacterial and viral infections long before AIDS. The first condoms date back to the 19th century, when they were used for disease prevention more often than contraception (Katchadourian, 1987). Sexually transmitted HIV infection, however, led to a 60% increase in U.S. condom sales between 1987 and 1989, with more than 450 million condoms sold each year in the United States alone (Consumer Reports, 1995). Condoms are now manufactured from a number of different materials, including latex of varying thickness and textures, natural membranes, and polyurethane. Female condoms or vaginal liners are another optional barrier method. Although condoms are well known to reduce risks for STDs, their relative effectiveness for preventing HIV transmission has been the subject of considerable scrutiny.

Male Condoms

Several studies have tested the efficacy of latex condoms in protecting against HIV transmission. Latex is impermeable to herpes simplex virus and cytomegalovirus, both of which are smaller in size than sperm and bacteria, but larger than HIV (Feldblum & Fortney, 1988). Therefore, when first considering latex condoms as a prophylactic against HIV infection, it was not possible to rely solely on previous research that determined condoms protect against other STDs.

Condom efficacy studies fall into two categories: in-vitro studies that test the permeability of latex in laboratory settings and in-vivo studies that test condom performance during sexual intercourse. In-vitro studies typically inflate various brands of condoms with water or air and test their burst and/or leakage potential under pressure. Although valuable data are obtained, these studies do not speak to the diffusion of HIV across pores of stretched but intact latex. Laboratory research on condom efficacy has shown that latex condoms vary in their ability to contain HIV, but latex condoms consistently reduce risks for HIV transmission. An early study of latex permeability placed highly concentrated solutions of mouse retrovirus and HIV inside three latex condoms and two types of nonlatex condoms. This study found that virus particles did not leak across to the tissue medium (Conant, Hardy, Sernatinger, Spicer, & Levy, 1986). It is important to note, however, that this study used a passive test of HIV leakage across intact membranes and does not speak to viral transfer when latex is stretched or challenged by heat and friction, both of which occur during intercourse.

In a rigorous test of the limits of latex condom effectiveness for HIV prevention, Carey, Herman, Retta, Rinaldi, and Herman (1992) challenged latex condoms with 30 minutes of stretching over a penile form to simulate stretching that occurs when condoms are worn during intercourse. Following the stretching, Carey et al. injected a solution into the tip of the condom through the penile form to simulate ejaculation. The fluid injected into the condom was of a viscosity more like water than semen, providing a more likely medium for leakage. The injected fluid contained fluorescence labeled microspheres that approximated the size of HIV (110 nanometers) and the fluid was left in the stretched condom for 10 minutes. The study found that 29 of 89 condoms tested did leak virus-sized particles. However, even in the worst case of leakage, it was estimated that condoms provided 10,000 times greater protection against exposure to HIV during sexual intercourse than would no use of condoms. Results of other in-vitro studies are similar and lead to the same conclusion: that intact latex condoms effectively protect against HIV transmission.

In-vivo studies typically involve couples with one partner who is HIV infected and the other who is not (serodiscordant couples) to observe whether condoms protect against HIV transmission. These studies have consistently shown that latex condoms protect against HIV infection. For example, Saracco et al. (1993) prospectively studied HIV-seronegative women who were in stable, monogamous relationships with HIV-infected men and found that among the women whose partners consistently used condoms during sexual intercourse, only three (2%) contracted HIV, compared to eight of 55 (15%) women who reported inconsistent condom use. The rate of HIV infection was 7.2 per 100 women per year who did not consistently use condoms and 1.1 women per 100 who did consistently use condoms. Similar findings were reported by De Vincenzi (1994) in a study of heterosexual serodiscordant couples, where none of the couples that reported consistent use of condoms over the course of 15,000 sex acts experienced HIV transmission compared to 10% of those who inconsistently used condoms. In yet another study, Diaz, Chu, Conti, Sorvillo, and Cheko (1994) interviewed heterosexually HIV-infected persons and found that 1% always used condoms and 29% never used condoms during intercourse during the 5 years before they became infected. The study found that 35% of infected women had only one sex partner in the 5 years before they became infected, and these women were the least likely to use condoms during intercourse. These findings are compelling and support laboratory studies that show latex condoms effectively prevent HIV transmission.

Latex condoms are inexpensive, widely available, and often recommended for both contraception and disease prevention. However, not all condoms are made of latex. Condoms made from natural membranes, most commonly lamb intestines, are durable and increase the sensation of sexual stimulation during intercourse. Increased sensitivity of natural membrane condoms results from pores in the membranes that allow fluids to flow in and out. These pores are nearly half the width of sperm, making natural membranous condoms a viable contraceptive. However, as noted earlier, natural condoms offer minimal protection against viral transmission because viruses, including HIV, are many times smaller than sperm.

Another alternative to latex condoms are those made of a soft, durable plastic that is not susceptible to deterioration caused by oils or poor storage conditions. Polyurethane is thinner than latex and allows for greater transfer of heat, suggesting that they may be more acceptable, particularly among people who are allergic to latex (approximately 3% of the population) or those who are dissatisfied with latex condoms (Trussell, Warner, & Hatcher, 1992a). Research has shown that polyurethane is an effective barrier against transmitting HIV and other STDs. Responses to polyurethane condoms have been generally positive in marketing research (Rosenberg, Waugh, Solomon, & Lyszkowski, 1996). However, because polyurethane does not stretch, men with larger than average penises may find them uncomfortable and men with smaller than average penises may experience greater slippage during intercourse (Consumer Reports, 1995). Thus, although more expensive and less proven than latex condoms, polyurethane condoms are a viable option for preventing sexually transmitted HIV infections.

Condom Failure

Condoms fail when they are not used properly or when they leak, break, tear, or slip off. A national survey found that 13% of men who use condoms experience breaks or tears, and 14% had condoms slip off during sexual intercourse (Grady, Klepinger, Billy, & Tanfer, 1993). The majority of heterosexual couples who consistently use condoms experience breaks at some point (Hatcher & Hughes, 1988). Studies that enroll couples who use condoms or are instructed to use condoms have found a wide range of condom performances. Condom breakage rates in prospective studies where couples are asked to use various brands of latex condoms have ranged between nearly perfect performance (.5% breakage) to moderate failure rates (6.7%, Albert, Warner, Hatcher, Trussell, & Bennett, 1995). Condoms slip off during intercourse or while withdrawing the penis after ejaculation, at rates that vary from .6% to 5.4% of condom uses (Albert et al., 1995). Overall, latex condoms fail due to breakage or slippage approximately 2% to 5% of the time (Trussell, Hatcher, Cates, Stewart, & Kost, 1990). Much of the variability in condom performance is accounted for by factors such as differences in vaginal or anal lubrication, penis size, width of vaginal or anal opening, and other anatomically and physiologically related individual differences. Latex has a limited shelf life, approximately 3 years when properly stored (Consumer Reports, 1995), so the age of latex condoms can be a significant factor in their ability to remain intact during intercourse (Steiner et al., 1994). Latex condoms, however, are practically doomed to failure when used with oil-based lubricants. Oil-containing lubricants, even if water soluble, quickly degrade latex condoms, making them porous and brittle. Only oil-free, water-based products should therefore be used to lubricate latex condoms. The improper use of oil-containing lubricants is common, however, with 60% of homosexually active men reporting use of oil-containing products, including hand lotions and baby oils, during anal intercourse (Martin, 1992).

Condom failures vary during vaginal, anal, and oral intercourse. Condoms break and slip off at higher rates during anal intercourse than vaginal intercourse (Trussell, Warner, & Hatcher, 1992b), and condoms rarely fail during oral intercourse (Thompson, Yager, & Martin, 1993). Among heterosexuals, 3.4% report condoms breaking and 1.1% report condoms slipping off during their most recent sexual intercourse occasion (Messiah, Dart, Spencer, & Warszawski, 1997). Condom failure is common among gay men who practice anal intercourse. Ross (1987) reported that 14% of gay men in Australia experienced a few breaks and 13% reported many condom breaks during anal intercourse. Another study of gay men found 31% experienced condom breaks at least once during anal intercourse (Golombok, Sketchley, & Rust, 1989). Research with over 500 male sex workers in San Francisco showed that 58% experienced condom breaks and 47% had condoms slip off, with most failures occurring during anal intercourse (Waldorf & Lauderback, 1993). Thompson et al. (1993) reported that overall condom breakage rates during a single episode of receptive anal intercourse were 2.7% compared to 3.3% for insertive anal intercourse. In an Australian sample, condoms broke during 5.1% of receptive anal intercourse occasions compared to 7.3% of insertive acts (Tindall, Swanson, Donovan, & Cooper, 1989). Given that differences between receptive and insertive anal intercourse are based on self-reports gathered from receptive and insertive partners, respectively, it is possible that insertive partners are more aware of condom performance during intercourse and may not always inform their partners of the problem. Supporting this conclusion is a survey conducted with gay and bisexual men that found 12% of men who experienced condom breakage/slippage during anal intercourse had not informed their partner of the failure (Kalichman, Schaper, Belcher, Abush–Kirsh, & Cherry, 1997).

Another factor known to influence condom failure is the past experience of the individual using the condom. Proper use of condoms requires both application before intercourse starts and continuous use of condoms during the entire duration of intercourse. As many as half of men report removing condoms after initiating intercourse at least once and 17% do so repeatedly (Richters, Gerofi, & Donovan, 1993). Condoms are more prone to burst when air bubbles remain between the latex and penis, either in the tip of the condom or along the shaft. Condoms can also tear while putting them on from pinching with fingernails or piercing with jewelry. More frequent use of condoms is associated with greater success. Thompson et al. (1993) found that gay men in a New York City cohort where significantly less likely to experience condom breaks if they had previous experience using condoms. For men who had not previously used condoms during receptive anal intercourse, 15% reported condom failure during the one time they did use a condom. This rate fell to 1.5% for men who had used condoms four or five times before, and to less than 1% for those who used condoms 10 or more times. Thompson et al. concluded that men who have only used condoms once or twice should exercise particular care until they gain more experience. Similarly, Albert et al. (1995) reported the lowest rates of condom failure in the literature among commercial sex workers. Female commercial sex workers who used condoms during every act of vaginal intercourse did so without a single condom breakage. Thus, proficient use of condoms gained from experience leads to increased success, and reduces frustrations with condoms that could lead to discontinued use. Condom failure among experienced users therefore occurs much less frequently than among less experienced users (Messiah et al., 1997). The benefits of experience using condoms also supports the value of experiential training and practice sessions in using condoms during prevention interventions.

Female Condoms

Until recently, condom use was entirely dependent on a man's willingness to put one on his penis. However, a female-controlled method of barrier protection was approved for use and made available in 1993. The female condom is made of polyurethane, the same soft, light, plastic material described earlier. The female condom is a loose-fitting pouch with two flexible rings; one that remains inside the bottom of the condom to serve as an insertion device and an internal anchor, and another ring at the top that remains outside the vagina to protect the labia and base of the penis. Figure 2.1 shows the Reality® female condom and instructions for its proper use. The female condom is an effective contraceptive and disease prevention option (Farr, Gabelnick, Sturgen, & Dorflinger, 1994; Soper et al., 1993). There is an overall estimated 26% failure rate for pregnancy, and the failure rate is 11% when used consistently and correctly (CDC, 1993). The efficacy of female condoms in protection against HIV infection, however, has been less well documented. Consumer research has shown that women like the idea of a female condom because it affords them control in health decisions (Shervington, 1993). However, as with many things new, unfamiliarity with female condoms has made them awkward to use and easy to misuse. Female condoms are also several times more expensive than latex male condoms. Thus, state governments and insurance providers started paying for female condoms. The female condom has also become popular among gay and bisexual men for use during anal intercourse, although female condoms used for anal intercourse are of unknown safety and effectiveness.

Condom Attitudes and Perceptions

The potential for condoms to prevent sexually transmitted HIV infection is offset by the resistance of people to consistently use condoms. National

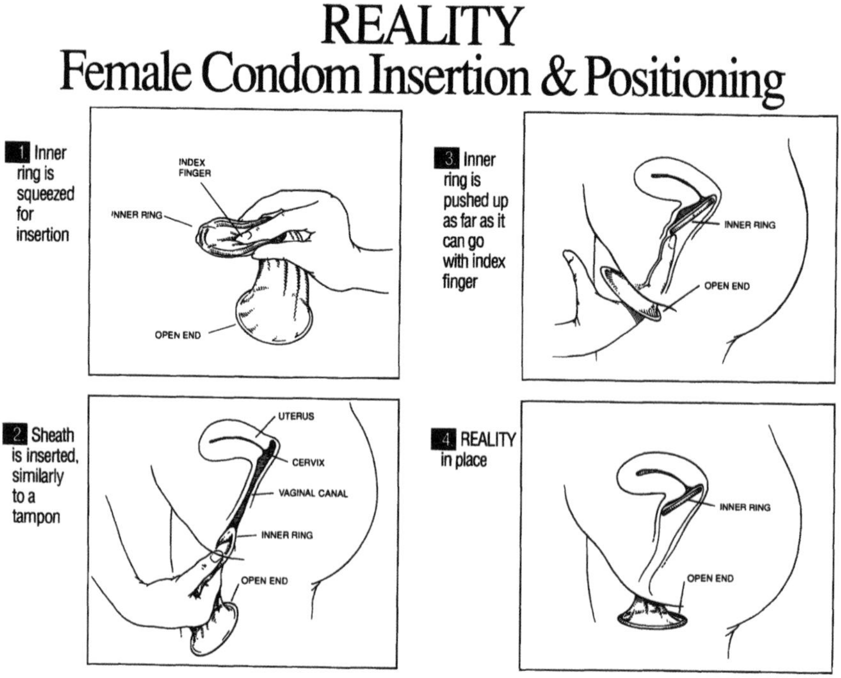

REALITY
Female Condom Insertion & Positioning

FIG. 2.1. The Reality® condom and the steps for its proper use.

surveys show that nearly two thirds of sexually active men do not use condoms at all during sexual intercourse (Tanfer et al., 1993). Women living in inner cities with high-risk behavior histories are no more likely to use condoms than are women at lower behavioral risk, with less than half of all vaginal intercourse occasion protected by condoms (Kalichman, Hunter, & Kelly, 1992). Among homosexually active men, Kelly et al. (1992) reported that men who engaged in unprotected anal intercourse had no intention to use condoms in the future. Condom use is also infrequent among injection drug users, with nearly half of men who inject drugs never using condoms with their steady sex partners and half never using them with casual partners (CDC, 1992). A national survey found that almost one third of African American adults do not use condoms with either primary or casual sex partners (Grinstead, Peterson, Faigeles, & Catania, 1997). Although people with multiple sex partners are more likely to use condoms than are those in long-standing relationships, long-term partners often confer considerable risks for HIV infection (Upchurch, Ray, Reichart, Celentano, & Quinn, 1992).

There are many reasons why people refuse to use condoms. When considered for contraception, condoms are less effective and more inconvenient than other available methods. Nevertheless, condoms are the only contraceptive method that also offer protection against STDs. Still, few women who use other methods of contraception also use condoms for STD protection. For example, Santelli, Davis, Celentano, Crump, and Burwell (1995) found that 62% of women on the pill also used condoms and this was a significantly greater rate of condom use than observed among women who used other contraceptive methods. Condoms are also not used in relationships that are perceived as safe. Condoms are least likely used in relationships that are labeled steady or exclusive, and condom use is likely discontinued as relationships progress (Kippax, Crawford, Davis, Rodden, & Dowsett, 1993; Misovich, Fisher, & Fisher, in press).

Characteristics of condoms themselves are also known to reduce the likelihood of their use. Negative attitudes toward condoms have significantly predicted their use among men (O'Donnell, Doval, Duran, & O'Donnell, 1995), women (Valdiserri, Arena, Proctor, & Bonati,1989), and adolescents (DiClemente et al., 1992; Pendergrast, DuRant, & Gaillard, 1992). In Australia, 68% of homosexually active men reported that condoms reduced sensitivity during anal intercourse, which in turn reduced the likelihood that they would use them during sex (Ross, 1987, 1992). Other negative experiences adversely impact condom use, including experiences with breakage and slippage during intercourse and loss of erection during condom use.

Condom attitudes encompass individual beliefs about the efficacy, acceptability, accessibility, and value of condoms in preventing STDs. Condoms are often believed to disrupt the natural flow of sex, interrupt foreplay, and reduce pleasure. Condoms can also literally interrupt sex by interfering with erection. For example, the majority of men in a large Australian study reported at least partial loss of their erection after putting on a condom (Richters et al., 1995), a finding that replicates earlier research (Golombok, Sketchley, & Rust, 1989). Interference with the ability to gain and maintain an erection may result from disrupted sex play, reduced stimulation, as well as the association that condoms have with images of disease, AIDS, and death. The use of condoms can communicate a sense of mistrust or infidelity to sex partners. Survey data from over 5,000 heterosexual adults showed that 37% worried about losing their partner's trust by suggesting the use of condoms (Choi, Rickman, & Catania, 1994). Additional research has shown that women fear initiating condom use because they believe their partners would leave them or abuse them for suggesting condom use (Kalichman & Stevenson, 1997; Rothenberg & Paskey, 1995). Thus, trust and care in loving relationships can paradoxically reduce condom use and increase risk for STDs and HIV infection.

Condom attitudes are best described as an individual's beliefs about condoms and their use. Factor analytic studies have demonstrated reliable dimensions that capture a variety of facets of condom attitudes. For example, in a study of homosexually active men, Ross (1988) identified five condom attitude dimensions: (1) condoms as unreliable and antierotic; (2) condoms as offering protection from infection; (3) availability of condoms; (4) condoms interrupt sex play; and (5) experience of responsibility and comfort using condoms. Similarly, Chapman, Stoker, Ward, Porritt, and Fahey (1990) surveyed bisexually active persons and found three condom attitudinal factors: (1) using condoms as a positive action; (2) embarrassment obtaining and using condoms; and (3) condoms as antithetical to satisfying sex. In research with heterosexual college students, Sacco, Levine, Reed, and Thompson (1991) identified eight condom attitudinal dimensions: (1) interpersonal impact; (2) effect on sexual experience; (3) self-control; (4) global attitudes; (5) perceived risk; (6) inhibition; (7) promiscuity; and (8) relationship safety. Studies of adolescents using a similar but briefer instrument derived from Sacco et al.'s item pool demonstrated similar condom attitude factors (St. Lawrence et al., 1994). Additional factor analytic research has identified similar dimensions reflecting discomfort, interruption of sex, acceptability, inconvenience, and reduced pleasure (Johnson, Hinkle, Gilbert, & Gant, 1992).

In addition to negative perceptions that create barriers to using condoms, a number of other factors interfere with motivation to use condoms. In their research with women, Hobfoll, Jackson, Lavin, Britton, and Shepherd (1994) identified four principle barriers to condom use in addition to negative condom attitudes: (1) objections by sex partners to use condoms; (2) perceptions of personal risk for HIV infection, including perceptions of partner's past sexual history; (3) loss of sexual pleasure; and (4) embarrassment about sex in general and embarrassment about condom use in particular. Perceived barriers hamper motivations and intentions to use condoms. Condom barriers, including negative attitudes, vary across sexual relationships, partnerships, and situations. Thus, overcoming condom barriers requires attention to the unique properties of an individual's sexual risk-producing situations. The failure of many individuals to use condoms and the need for female-controlled methods for HIV and STD prevention has led to the search for alternative methods for preventing HIV transmission.

SAFER SEX

The term *safe sex* was coined for the AIDS epidemic and has become absorbed into Western culture. By definition, safe sex is a class of behaviors that confer no risk for HIV infection; sex partners do not exchange blood, semen, or vaginal secretions. Any sexual act that does not potentially expose a person to HIV is therefore deemed safe. Only nonpenetrative sexual behaviors such as hugging, holding, kissing, touching, massage, and the like qualify as safe sex practices unless, of course, both partners are known to be HIV negative, in which case safety is a given. An underlying assumption in HIV prevention, however, is that once people begin engaging in sexual intercourse they are not likely to stop. Safe sex is therefore only considered a viable outcome for prevention efforts targeted to young persons, particularly adolescents, who may delay engaging in sexual intercourse and restrict their sexual activity to nonpenetrative acts. For the most part, HIV prevention interventions target safer sex practices such as reduced risks offered by condom use or switching from the highest risk behaviors (unprotected anal and vaginal intercourse) to lower risk behaviors (oral sex).

Safer sex is defined by sexual activities that significantly reduce but do not eliminate risks for HIV infection, such as is the case of condom use during anal and vaginal intercourse. Increased condom use is one universally accepted goal of HIV prevention efforts. Definitions of safer sex have also included oral–genital contact (Ostrow et al., 1995), but the safety of oral sex has been controversial. Withdrawal before ejaculation can also be considered safer than intercourse to ejaculation (De Vincenzi, 1994), but because pre-ejaculatory fluids contain HIV and because many men fail to withdraw before ejaculation, withdrawal is of questionable safety. Safer sex therefore has several definitions and is ultimately determined by community and individual standards. Various HIV prevention programs therefore define a variety of sexual behaviors as safer. The following excerpts from brochures and pamphlets distributed for HIV prevention illustrate how communities have defined safer sex.

> Safer sex means keeping the fluids which carry HIV (blood, semen, and vaginal fluids) outside you and your partner's body. Latex condoms are your best way to prevent the exchange of these fluids. Think about it. Unsafe sex may seem hot in the moment, but practicing safer sex may save your life in the long run. Practicing safer sex is the best way to show your respect for each other.

> Holding another man, rubbin' against his body, jackin' off together or lickin' him ... these are just some of the ways you and your partner can express your desire and still be safer. Anything that doesn't let blood, semen, or vaginal fluids inside your body is completely safe. Use your imagination and find ways to have safer sex.

> Figure out for yourself what you will and will not do sexually. Draw a line on risk and stick to it. Commit to a safe level for you and your partner(s). There's nothing better than knowing that the sex you had before was great fun and safe.

> *Safer sex means being smart and staying healthy. It means showing love, concern, and respect for your partner and yourself .... Safer sex doesn't have to mean eliminating sexual passion and intimacy from your life. Safer sex means reducing the chance of acquiring HIV infection. For individuals who decide to engage in sexual intercourse, reducing risk for HIV infection means using latex condoms every time you have intercourse.*

Safer sex messages are also tailored to particular sexual preferences or tastes, as illustrated in the following excerpt from a brochure appealing to men involved in leather, bondage, and related activities: "Imagine being bound while a hot man rubs his leather clad pouch in your face ... safer sex doesn't mean vanilla. SAFER IS HOT!" The variety of interpretations of safer sex is important to understanding HIV prevention messages and expected outcomes from risk reduction interventions. Behavioral definitions of risk reduction, such as rates of condom use, frequencies of protected intercourse, and ratios of protected sex partners and protected acts offer greater precision for measuring changes in risk levels compared to broad constructs such as safer sex. Similarly, prevention messages that call for safer sex without defining safety in behavioral terms remain open to interpretation and could reinforce engaging in risky practices that are erroneously believed to be safer.

SEXUAL COMMUNICATION

All efforts to prevent sexually transmitted HIV infection occur in the context of interpersonal, intimate relationships. A major element of HIV prevention interventions therefore involves working toward increasing an individual's abilities to communicate assertively and effectively with sex partners. Sexual assertiveness includes initiating wanted or desired sexual activities, refusing unwanted sexual activities, and discussing or insisting on using condoms (Grimley, Prochaska, & Prochaska, 1993). HIV risk-reduction communication can include initiating discussions about sexual needs and desires, HIV antibody testing, safer sex, and condom use. Communicating about condom use may be particularly important for men who engage in receptive anal intercourse and for women because they must assure that their partners wear condoms. Unfortunately, lack of experience and confidence in discussing sex with partners interferes with initiating safer sex discussions. For example, women at risk for HIV infection often find it difficult to discuss condoms with sex partners, do not feel confident that they can persuade sex partners to use condoms, and believe that men can easily persuade them to have sex without condoms even when they really do not want to (Sikkema, Koob, Cargill, Kelly, Desiderato et al., 1995; Wingood & DiClemente, 1992). Women, particularly women living in poverty, tend to be in power-imbalanced relationships where they experience little control over their sexual interactions and feel ineffective at getting men to wear condoms. Similarly, gay men experience difficulties requesting that their sex partners use condoms and negotiate safety in their sexual relationships (Kippax et al., 1993). Gay and bisexual men also experience coercion to engage in unprotected anal intercourse, indicating a lack of assertiveness to refuse and resist partner pressure for unsafe sex (Kalichman & Rompa, 1995).

Aside from simply requesting condom use, sexual communication can also include a broader discussion of issues related to sexual health. Partners may discuss their sexual pasts and gain better understanding of each other's histories. They may also discuss HIV-antibody testing and the option of getting tested together. Once they test HIV seronegative together, a couple may negotiate safety in their relationship, such as by not using condoms with each other and remaining monogamous. Couples may also agree to practice safer sex with other partners if they choose not to be monogamous. Negotiated safety, however, is complicated by the fact that people are often dishonest in their relationships. For example, one survey found that HIV seropositive men often do not disclose their serostatus to sex partners, and that a significant number of men report lying about their sexual histories (Cochran & Mays, 1990). The potential lack of honesty in sexual relationships, the common experience of brief serial monogamy, and infidelities in relationships make negotiated safety an uncertain risk reduction option. Thus, sexual communication must be placed in the realm of other risk reduction strategies, but unlike abstinence and condom use, sexual communication relies on assumptions of partner openness and honesty.

HIV RISK REDUCTION THEORY

HIV transmission and the behaviors that reduce HIV transmission risks are determined by individual actions. Because the HIV epidemic is driven by behavior, psychological and social theories of human behavior and behavior change have made enormous contributions to the design, development, and evaluation of HIV risk-reduction interventions. Built on cognitive–attitudinal and affective–motivational constructs, theories of behavior change have been instrumental in identifying correlates of change that are capable of being articulated in instructional activities and included in HIV risk-reduction programs. The following sections briefly describe behavior-change theories that have most influenced and guided the advancement of HIV prevention interventions.

Health Belief Model

The health belief model was first developed in the 1950s as a means of explaining individual responses to illness symptoms, diagnoses, treatment, and the reasons why people do not participate in public health interventions and medical programs (Rosenstock, Strecher, & Becker, 1994). The health belief model is grounded in traditional social psychology and is based on the premise that perceptions of personal threats are a necessary precursor to taking preventive action. As shown in Fig. 2.2, the health belief model has four

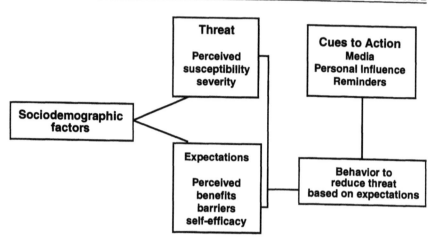

FIG. 2.2. The Health Belief Model

principle components: (1) individual differences that influence behavior; (2) perceived susceptibility and perceived severity of a health threat; (3) values or expectancies for taking action, including perceived benefits, barrier effectiveness, and costs for action; and (4) cues in the environment that promote action. Beliefs about threats of potential risks and outcome expectancies are thought to produce readiness for action, allowing beliefs to serve as causal agents for behavior. Thus, modifications of belief systems are posited to result in behavioral changes.

Subjective judgments of perceived susceptibility to a health threat and perceived severity of the threat are mediated by many factors. First, internal and external cues can trigger preventive action. Cues that may lead to protective behavior include internal states, such as bodily sensations, and environmental events including media messages or other sources of information (Rosenstock, Strecher, & Becker, 1994). Beliefs can also be mediated by sociodemographic characteristics, personality dispositions, and other individual difference factors. Research has suggested that the health belief model is applicable to HIV risk reduction where perceived vulnerability to AIDS, beliefs about the severity of AIDS, perceptions of risk-reducing actions, and environmental cues, such as knowing someone who is diagnosed with HIV infection or AIDS, correspond with an individual's interest in taking steps to reduce their personal risks.

Theory of Reasoned Action

Similar to the health belief model, the theory of reasoned action has its roots in traditional social psychology. Developed by Fishbein, the theory of reasoned action originated to explain human behavior and has been applied to a broad spectrum of health-related behaviors (Fishbein & Ajzen, 1975). In the theory of reasoned action, cognitive processes, particularly attitudes about behaviors and perceived norms for practicing behaviors, lead to intentions that are only one step away from engaging in a specific behavior (see Fig. 2.3). Behavioral intentions are themselves determined by attitudes, beliefs, and perceptions, all of which are influenced by social contexts and individual experiences. Attitudes and beliefs shared among members of a community, or social norms, serve as important social forces that influence intentions and behavior. Thus, behavior change is inherently connected to underlying attitude, belief, and perception structures (Fishbein, Middlestadt, & Hitchcock, 1994).

The theory of reasoned action emphasizes processes of behavior change, starting with specific definitions of target behaviors. Each behavior must be considered an independent entity with its own determinants, contingencies, and values. Specificity of behaviors and social systems must also be considered with reference to context and time (Fishbein et al., 1994). Precision in defining behaviors of interest is particularly important in this theory because specification of behavior allows one to identify intentions and delineate underlying attitudinal structures. Fishbein et al. (1994) described the implications of defining various behaviors, their contexts, and time as follows:

> That is, every action occurs with respect to some target, in a given context, and at a given point in time. Although one may arrive at more general behavioral criteria by generalizing across one or more of these elements, a change in any one of the four elements redefines the behavior of interest. For example, using a condom is a different behavior from carrying or buying a condom (a change in action); going to an STD clinic is a different behavior from going to a family doctor or going to a human immunodeficiency virus counseling and testing site (a change in target); using a condom with a spouse or long-term partner is a different behavior from using a condom with a casual partner or commercial sex worker (a change in context); and going to an STD clinic on a Tuesday morning is a different behavior from going to the same STD clinic on a Saturday

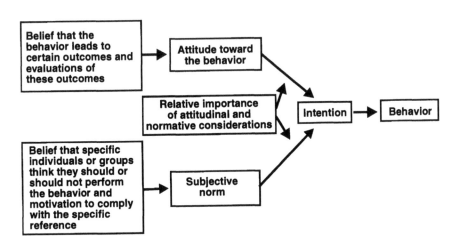

FIG. 2.3. The Theory of Reasoned Action.

afternoon (a change in time). It is worth noting that "using a condom the next time I have vaginal sex with my main partner" is a different behavior from "using a condom every time I have vaginal sex with my main partner" (p. 64).

Behavior is therefore a function of the deliberate processing of information available to the person in a given context at a given time. Behavior is determined by intentions, attitudes, perceived normative pressures, beliefs about consequences, values placed on perceived norms, and values placed on potential outcomes.

The theory of reasoned action is also based on the premise that behaviors are under the direct control of individuals as inferred by the volitional nature of intentions. However, there are many instances when individuals lack direct control over their actions, and the theory of reasoned action is limited in explaining behaviors under these circumstances. In response to this limitation, Ajzen (1988; Ajzen & Fishbein, 1980; Ajzen & Madden, 1986) developed the theory of planned behavior that states that perceived control constitutes a central construct in explaining behavior change. The theory of planned behavior states that under conditions when an individual either has limited control or perceives that he or she has limited control, these beliefs must be considered in addition to perceptions about the behavior, attitudes, norms, and intentions.

Social Cognitive Theory

Social cognitive theory is based on the premise that behaviors, environmental influences, attitudes, and beliefs are highly interactive and interdependent. As shown in Fig. 2.4, there is triadic reciprocal causation, or functional dependence, between behavior (B); intrapersonal factors including cognitive, affective, and biological processes (P); and the external environment (E). Social cognitive theory emphasizes the roles of outcome expectancies and reinforcement value for instituting behavior changes (Bandura, 1986, 1989, 1994). Central to social cognitive theory, however, are self-efficacy beliefs, defined as "one's capabilities to organize and execute the courses of action required to produce given attainments" (Bandura, 1997, p. 3). Self-efficacy is tied to performing specific actions under specified conditions and is therefore distinguished from outcome expectancies, self-esteem, and perceived control.

Social cognitive theory states that behavior change occurs as a direct result of observation and interpretation of behavioral performances. Processes involved in modeling and practicing specific behaviors are theorized to result in increased positive outcome expectancies, increased self-efficacy, and increased probability of receiving reinforcement for initial behavioral changes. Health-related behavior programs based on social cognitive theory generally target four interactive determinants of behavior (Bandura, 1994, 1997). First, behavior change requires accurate information to increase awareness and knowledge of risks associated with specific risk-producing practices. Second, individuals must possess social and self-management skills to allow effective action. Third, preventive behavior changes require enhancement of skills and

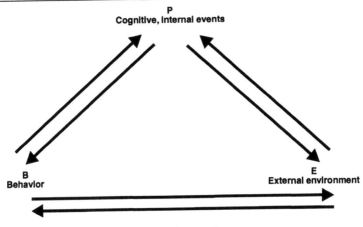

FIG. 2.4. Social Cognitive Theory.

the development of self-efficacy, usually accomplished through guided practice and corrective feedback on skill performance. Finally, behavior change entails creating social supports and reinforcements for behavior changes. Thus, interventions built on cognitive behavioral principles integrate information, attitude change to enhance motivation, development and reinforcement of risk reduction behavioral skills, and self-efficacy to implement changes in behavior.

Interventions based on social cognitive theory typically include four components: (1) risk education; (2) threat sensitization; (3) motivational enhancement to promote readiness to change; and (4) skills training that includes an initial explanation of new skills; modeling performance of the skills; discussion of strengths, weaknesses, and feasibility of the model's performance; and providing opportunities for practicing new skills with corrective feedback and social reinforcement for behavior change efforts (Bandura, 1986). These theoretical components are expressed in intervention exercises and activities. Individuals are provided with descriptions of effective behaviors, modeling the behavior by a person who shares characteristics with the intended target, and opportunities to practice the behavior with feedback on performance. Thus, activities are used to build behavioral skills and develop a sense of self-efficacy for performing new behaviors.

Transtheoretical Model

The transtheoretical model was developed as an overarching description of change processes that occur across a variety of behavioral domains (Prochaska, DiClemente, & Norcross, 1992). First developed from a comparative analysis of leading systems of psychotherapy, the stages of change model was designed to represent a continuum that spans from nonchange to readiness to change to taking action. The model proposes that people move through a sequence of change processes that are ordered by degrees of motivation and behavior (see Fig. 2.5). Precontemplation is the first stage in the change process, where an individual is not mindful of a potential problem and has no intention to change. The second stage, contemplation, occurs when an individual recognizes the need to change behavior and intends to make a change, followed by a preparatory, planning, ready-for-action stage. The next stage is defined by taking action steps to enact behavioral changes. Finally, there is a maintenance stage that is characterized by efforts to sustain accomplished behavioral changes. The model also accounts for potential lapses to earlier behavior patterns in the change process (Prochaska, Redding, Harlow, Rossi, & Velicer, 1994). Progressing through successive stages of change varies from individual to individual and varies for different behavioral changes.

The transtheoretical model offers a useful heuristic for describing behavior change. Like the theory of reasoned action and other models, the transtheoretical model emphasizes the primacy of cognitive processes. In fact, contemplating behavioral changes is operationalized by the transtheoretical model as intentions to change behavior (Prochaska et al., 1994). Progression through the stages of change is determined by cognitive–behavioral processes at each stage. Consciousness raising is the process that moves a person from precontemplation to contemplative stages; self-reevaluation moves one from contemplative to preparation and planning; and reinforcement management and stimulus control move individuals through action steps to behavior change maintenance. The transtheoretical model offers a wide range of targeted behavioral outcomes and suggests that an individual's present status in the change process should be considered when designing interventions. It is therefore possible to prescribe interventions matched to an individual's stage of readiness to change. Intervention strategies matched to stages of change

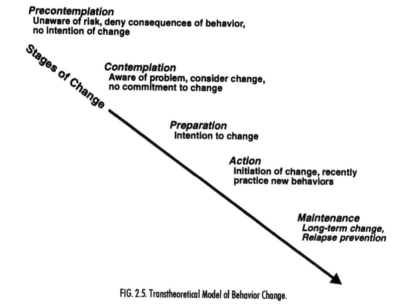

FIG. 2.5. Transtheoretical Model of Behavior Change.

move the person to the next stage until ultimately supporting maintenance of changed behavior. An intervention designed to move a person from the precontemplation stage to contemplative stage will therefore have expected outcomes related to awareness and conscientiousness, and outcomes from an intervention for people in the contemplative stage will enhance intentions to change, whereas behavior change is only a reasonable intervention outcome for individuals who are ready for action. The transtheoretical model has influenced the development of many HIV-risk education interventions, but it has also been criticized for its lack of theoretical specificity and conceptual clarity.

Models Specific to HIV Risk Reduction

Acknowledging both the contributions and limitations of generalized psychological theories of behavior change for HIV risk and risk reduction, there is a recognized need for models that specifically address the complexities of sexual behavior and drug use (Kelly & Kalichman, 1995). HIV prevention researchers have proposed models that are tailored to HIV risk and preventive behaviors. These models encompass many of the same constructs delineated by the health belief model, the theory of reasoned action, social cognitive theory, and the transtheoretical model. However, HIV-risk reduction models offer greater specificity for HIV-preventive behaviors. Two models that have been derived for HIV risk reduction are the AIDS risk reduction model (ARRM; Catania, Kegeles, & Coates, 1990), and the information, motivation, behavioral skills model (IMB; Fisher & Fisher, 1992).

AIDS Risk Reduction Model. The ARRM was developed as a conceptual framework to organize behavior change factors related to HIV risk reduction. Using constructs derived from the health belief model, social cognitive theory, diffusion theory, and models of help seeking and decision making, ARRM constitutes a hybrid model crafted specifically for HIV prevention. ARRM is also a stage model, where an individual progresses through processes of behavior change (see Fig. 2.6). First, as derived from the health belief and the transtheoretical models, an individual must recognize and label their vulnerability for HIV infection. Once self-labeled as potentially vulnerable, a person is capable of making a commitment to changing their behavior, which can include changes in condom attitudes and gaining self-efficacy to use condoms. The final stage in the model is enactment, defined as the summation of labeling, commitment, and help seeking. In this sense, help seeking includes gaining support for changing risk behaviors, communicating with sex partners about change, and initiating condom use. ARRM therefore reconstructs previously articulated theoretical constructs to specifically apply to HIV risk reduction.

Information–Motivation–Behavioral Skills Model. In another model derived to explain HIV risk reduction behavior, Fisher and Fisher (1992) proposed a three-factor conceptualization of AIDS-preventive behavior:

information, motivation, and behavioral skills (see Fig. 2.7). The IMB model states that information about modes of HIV transmission and methods of preventing transmission is a necessary precursor to risk-reduction behavior. Motivation to change also directly affects whether one acts on information about risk and risk reduction. Finally, the model holds that behavioral skills related to preventive actions are a common pathway for information and motivation to result in AIDS preventive behavior change. The IMB model assumes that information and motivation activate behavioral skills to ultimately enact risk reduction behaviors. The model also shows that information or motivation alone can have direct effects on preventive behavior, such as when information about HIV transmission prompts purchasing condoms, or when meeting someone with HIV infection motivates a person to seek HIV antibody testing. Behavioral skills become increasingly important when preventive actions require complex skills, such as initiating condom use or discussing getting tested with a sex partner. The IMB is therefore constructed from elements found in previous theories, but configured specifically for HIV risk reduction. A strength of the IMB is its parsimony and specificity; packaging several constructs in three primary factors. Another strength of the IMB model is that its derivation was a product of conceptual analyses of successful HIV risk reduction interventions, providing a direct link between the model and intervention development. The IMB is among the most testable models in the HIV-prevention literature. Using path analyses, Fisher and Fisher (1992) illustrated that information, motivation, and behavioral skills predict risk-reduction behavioral outcomes. In addition, the IMB provides a useful heuristic for describing intervention components that are common to behavior change interventions based on most generalized theories of behavior change.

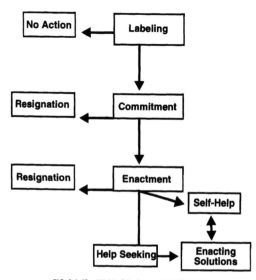

FIG. 2.6. The AIDS Risk Reduction Model (ARRM).

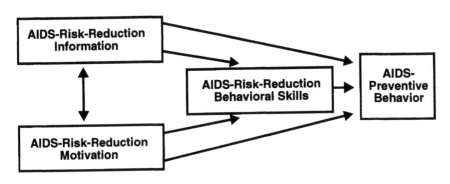

FIG. 2.7. The Information—Motivation—Behavioral Skills (IMB) Model

Summary of Formal Theories and Models

Four prominent theoretical formulations of behavior change have influenced HIV prevention efforts; the health belief model, the theory of reasoned action, social cognitive theory, and the transtheoretical model. These theories share several commonalities, including perceptions of threat and susceptibility, attitudes toward performing risk-reduction behaviors, normative beliefs about one's peers and community members, beliefs and attitudes about one's own ability to carry out preventive actions, the acquisition of social and behavioral skills that result in risk reduction, and motivational factors that bring a person to a state of readiness to act. As shown in Table 2.1, social and behavioral theories package principles of behavior change into various constructs and posit different mechanisms of behavior change. However, it can be seen that preventive interventions based on any of these components could be described by more than one of the models. Thus, what distinguishes the four major theories is which mechanisms and determinants they emphasize. But how the theoretical constructs are played out in HIV prevention interventions are far more similar than different. Prevention interventions may therefore emphasize perceptions of threat (health belief model), intentions to act (theory of reasoned action), self-efficacy to perform specific behavioral skills (social cognitive theory), or becoming motivated or ready to change (transtheoretical model). HIV risk-reduction interventions, however, reflect many of these elements that are common across theories (Fisher & Fisher, 1992; Kalichman, Carey, & Johnson, 1996).

Although the four theories described have been the most predominantly discussed in the HIV-prevention literature, they are not the only theories that have influenced HIV risk-reduction interventions. Theories of social networks (Needle, Coyle, Genser, & Trotter, 1995), behavioral decision making (Janis & Mann, 1977), and conservation of coping resources (Hobfoll, 1989) have played important roles in developing HIV risk-reduction interventions. Theories of social influence, social marketing (Ling, Franklin, Lindsteadt, &

TABLE 2.1
Theoretical Constructs Explaining Individual Behavior Change

Theory	Primary Constructs	Mechanism of Change
Health Belief Model (Rosenstock, Strecher, & Becker, 1994)	Individual; sociodemographic characteristics; threat perceptions; expectancies for benefits and barriers to action; cues to promote action	Beliefs concerning one susceptibility to risk exceed threshold to trigger taking action to reduce risks
Theory of Reasoned Action (Fishbein & Ajzen, 1975)	Attitudes toward behavior; subjective norms; values associated with norms; behavioral intentions	Attitudinal changes lead to intentions to perform risk-reducing actions
Social Cognitive Theory (Bandura, 1986)	Reciprocal determinism among cognitive/affective; behavior; and environmental factors	Self-efficacy to perform risk-reducing behaviors in vulnerable situations
Transtheoretical Model (Prochaska & DiClemente, 1992)	Stages of change processes; precontemplation; contemplative; determination; action, maintenance; and relapse	Moving through stages of readiness to action

Gearon, 1992), and group processes have also influenced HIV prevention interventions (Winett, Altman, & King, 1990). For example, Rogers' (1995b) social diffusion theory has been the basis for a number of interventions that recruit influential opinion leaders in communities to serve as credible behavior change agents (Winett et al., 1995). Diffusion of innovations occurs through dynamic processes that unfold over time, and HIV risk-reduction behaviors themselves can be conceptualized as diffusing through social networks and ultimately impacting large numbers of persons and entire communities. For this reason, social diffusion theory has been attractive to HIV prevention efforts that are designed to influence populations and communities.

A major limitation of most theories used to guide HIV prevention interventions, however, is their lack of specificity to sexual desire, pleasure, affection, and sexual self-esteem. Although HIV prevention efforts recognize the critical role of human sexuality in behaviors driving the epidemic, the absence of a comprehensive theory of human sexual behavior has led to the adoption of health promotion, social action, and behavior change theories in HIV prevention interventions (Kelly & Kalichman, 1995). Relationships are at the core of sexually transmitted HIV infection, but the unique features of these relationships, including love, affection, self-esteem, power, survival, intimacy, coercion, lust, and trust, are not directly addressed by existing models of HIV-risk behavior change.

CONCLUSIONS

Risk for HIV infection is conferred by only a few specific behaviors and, therefore, only a few steps are necessary to prevent the sexual transmission of HIV. Sexually transmitted HIV can be avoided by abstaining from fluid exchanging sexual behaviors or by placing a barrier between infected fluids and susceptible cells. These few behaviors constitute the expected behavioral outcomes of HIV risk-reduction interventions. The apparent simplicity of HIV risk reduction is, of course, deceptive. The complexity of HIV risk-associated behaviors, their inextricable association with human relationships, and the private nature of targeted outcome behaviors make designing and evaluating the efficacy and effectiveness of HIV prevention interventions an enterprise faced with enormous challenges. As will be shown in upcoming chapters, great strides have, however, occurred in efforts to reduce HIV risk-related behaviors.

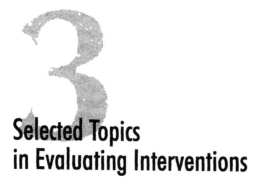

Selected Topics in Evaluating Interventions

HIV prevention ultimately hinges on the decisions and actions of individuals. Prevention interventions therefore seek to influence decisions and persuade people to take preventive actions. The success of an intervention is judged on the basis of its ability to reduce risk-related behaviors and decrease HIV transmission. This chapter examines the challenges encountered in designing and evaluating HIV prevention interventions. Although the majority of HIV prevention activities take place in public health clinics and community-based organizations, the focus here is on interventions implemented in the context of experimental and quasi-experimental HIV prevention studies. An exhaustive discussion of methodological issues relevant to HIV risk-reduction intervention research is beyond the scope of this chapter, and such resources are available elsewhere (e.g., Mantell, DiVittis, & Auerbach, 1997; Ostrow & Kessler, 1993). This overview provides a context for later discussions of the intervention outcome literature, specifically related to defining the roles of behavioral theory and community values in developing and designing HIV risk-reduction interventions, consideration of intervention format and delivery, and barriers to evaluating HIV prevention interventions.

INTERVENTION DESIGN ISSUES

Early in the HIV epidemic there was hope that behavioral interventions could be designed to affect a large mass of people to curtail the epidemic, or at least temporarily stop new HIV infections until a preventive vaccine became available. Time has shown that there is no quick fix that will stop the spread of

HIV and that developing HIV prevention technologies is an evolving process. Early HIV prevention interventions were void of theoretical principles, and this was true both of interventions conducted through community-based organizations and in prevention research (Fisher & Fisher, 1992). Formal theories of behavior change first influenced HIV prevention interventions in the late 1980s. As intervention development became informed by social and behavioral theories, community involvement was also integrated into the design of prevention interventions. Behavioral theories drive much of the content of interventions, whereas information from communities directs the context of intervention components. Content and context are embedded in the structure of the intervention, which consists of the number of intervention contacts, intensity of contact, and intervention dosage. The following sections overview the roles of theory and community input in intervention development, the structure in which interventions occur, and the challenges of evaluating prevention programs.

Theoretical Behavior Change Principles

As discussed in chapter 2, the theories that have most influenced HIV prevention place an emphasis on cognitive factors to guide behavioral changes. It is therefore common for interventions to target negative attitudes toward condoms, perceptions of invulnerability, perceived control over contracting HIV, self-efficacy for performing risk-reducing behaviors, and perceived social norms for supporting safer sex. Theories that emphasize the importance of enhancing motivations to change risk behaviors also play important roles in prevention intervention development (Fisher & Fisher, 1992; Prochaska, DiClemente, & Norcross, 1992). Behavioral theories have guided interventions by providing explanatory frameworks for intervention components and the interpretations of their outcomes. Theory-based interventions express constructs in their activities, which can be measured as mediators of behavior change or as outcome variables in their own right.

Linkages between theory, intervention components, and targeted outcomes can be empirically tested using analytic techniques that evaluate the effects of theoretical constructs, or mediating variables, on behavioral changes. Mediation analyses use a variety of statistical techniques, including multiple regression, path analyses, and structural equation modeling, each providing insight into the effects of theoretically derived intervention activities on targeted outcomes (Kazdin, 1992; West, Aiken, & Todd, 1993). Mediation analyses are most meaningful when they stem from an intervention that was built on a well-specified theoretical model. Mediating variables are derived from theory-driven intervention components and require reliable measurement instruments. Directed by theory, paths are defined for linking intervention components, mediating variables, and targeted outcome behaviors. Mediation analyses in the intervention outcome literature report path coefficients to show the influence of theoretical constructs on intervention outcomes. For example, health belief model constructs, including perceived susceptibility and perceived severity of HIV, condom attitudes, perceived control, and self-efficacy have been empirically shown through path analyses to predict intentions to use condoms and frequency of condom use (Bryan, Aiken, & West, 1996).

Behavioral theories have also been useful in describing the components of existing community-based programs. Community programs often mirror theoretically derived interventions but without specific linkages to formal constructs and without the theoretical jargon used to describe their activities. For example, there appears to be little difference between the communication skills training components described in theory-based interventions and the role play activities used in many community based programs. Both research-based and community-based interventions ask participants to practice communication and safer sex negotiation skills. Interventions in the research literature are more likely based on explicit theories of behavior change whereas the theoretical foundations for community based interventions are implicit. Research-based interventions designed to articulate a theory include a closely knit set of principles expressed in intervention activities. In contrast, community based programs include an array of intervention activities selected for their fit with community values and needs. However, studies have not tested interventions grounded in explicit theories against those based on community decisions. There are also no tests for fidelity in HIV prevention implementation, so there are no grounds for judging the relative effects of interventions delivered in research protocols versus those delivered by communities.

Community Involvement

The role that community members play in the development and design of research based HIV prevention interventions has undergone dramatic change over the course of the AIDS epidemic. There is a history of researchers implementing HIV prevention projects in neighborhood settings with minimal input from communities. Researchers who come into impoverished neighborhoods wanting to study STDs and AIDS work in the shadow of the Tuskegee syphilis study and other examples of researchers exploiting communities. Although researchers have often sought the cooperation of community organizations and community members, these arrangements rarely result in researcher-community collaboration. Fisher and Fisher (1992) reported that most intervention studies conducted throughout the 1980s and early 1990s did not perform minimum activities to involve community members in designing interventions, such as by eliciting information about community norms, social perceptions, values, and cultural contexts through formative research. Community-based agencies may support a study and assist in its execution, reflecting a cooperative model found in the tradition of clinical research. Facilitated by funding initiatives and other pressures, collaborative models, where researchers and community agencies form partnerships to develop and test interventions together, are beginning to replace cooperative models.

Collaborative partnerships between researchers and community groups have long existed in community health and community psychology, both of which build coalitions between researchers and communities. However, there is a tension between the values of researchers and community members that creates many barriers to community-research collaborations. Research-based interventions must remain true to the theoretical principles on which they are built in order to provide a valid test of a preventive model. Adherence to a structured protocol over the course of a study is also vital to protecting the scientific integrity of intervention research. From a community perspective, however, the ever-changing needs and priorities of communities demand flexibility rather than constancy in delivering intervention activities. In order for collaboration to occur, researchers must develop interventions and intervention study designs that are both scientifically rigorous and responsive to community needs. The cost to the study is the potential variability that occurs in intervention conditions, reducing statistical power in the research design. On the other hand, responsive research will help build greater community trust and investment in the research enterprise, paying-off in successful recruitment, reduced attrition, greater follow-up rates, and support for future projects.

There are many roles for community members in the intervention research enterprise. Community Advisory Boards (CABs), for example, are often assembled by researchers to review aspects of interventions and research methodologies during their developmental phases. Community advisors who typically support the research agenda provide feedback on such things as marketing and recruitment strategies, measurement instruments, assessment procedures, intervention plans, and research protocols. However, CABs often play a superficial role in a project, only providing the appearance of community involvement. It is unusual to find a CAB included in the organizational plan for a study or to find support for a CAB in a research budget. Although researchers have successfully gained considerable cooperation for their work from communities, there are few examples of true collaborations in the HIV-prevention intervention literature, where researchers and community groups share in decision making, benefits of funding, ownership, and final products. Collaborations between researchers and community agencies will, however, become more common as research funding demands community partnerships and as community programs require evaluation of their programs. Thus, establishing mutual benefits in community–researcher collaborations helps all parties to overcome their differences and helps bridge the gap between prevention practice and prevention science.

Format and Delivery

Intervention structure, as defined by format and delivery, is independent of intervention content. The format of an intervention is defined as its infrastructure, including such characteristics as the number of intervention sessions, amount of contact time, sequential ordering of components, homogeneity/heterogeneity of target population, and cultural contextualization. The same intervention can therefore be delivered in many different forms, each of which varies in number of contacts, amount of time per contact, components, and targeted audiences.

A major gap in the HIV risk-reduction literature is the limited information available to guide decisions regarding intervention format. Contact time in behavioral interventions ranges between 4 and 30 hours, without evidence that longer interventions result in greater behavioral changes. Intervention components that are common across prevention programs are tailored to fit the culture and lives of the targeted audience. However, there remains a virtual vacuum of information to guide the customization of context in which interventions are delivered. Although intervention structure surely affects outcomes, research has not tested the effects of various structural elements.

Other issues of behavioral intervention format and delivery concern the importance of adherence to specified intervention procedures. As mentioned earlier, there are no parameters established for determining the degree to which a prevention intervention should be delivered with fidelity. Delivering intervention components in a specified protocol must be balanced against the flexibility required to meet consumer needs. Adherence to a study protocol versus providing services to the community represents a significant tension between researchers and community groups. Unfortunately, the degree to which interventions can tolerate divergence from protocols and procedures without threatening their potential for positive outcomes is unknown.

Intervention Dosage

Intervention dosage typically refers to the time allocated to a fixed set of intervention components. For example, an intervention that consists of four components, such as risk education, sensitization to personal risks, sexual communication skills exercises, and relapse prevention, can manipulate intervention dosage, delivering all four components in either a 2 hour or 6 hour period of time. The amount of time, therefore, is altered to define dose. In some cases, however, dosage can refer to the delivery of different intervention components over a fixed amount of time. For example, the amount of time an intervention takes can be held constant while altering the components to which a person is exposed and in what relative proportion. Unfortunately, such biomedical conceptualizations of dose do not fit well when applied to behavioral interventions. In behavioral interventions, the program components are confounded with time; 20 minutes of role playing differs from 5 minutes of role playing in terms of rapport, participant comfort, openness, and other relevant interpersonal factors that are affected by time and are not independent of the role-play activity itself. Thus, the question of how much intervention time is needed for a desired outcome remains open. Unlike medical interventions where there are possible toxic effects and the potential for overdose, greater amounts of behavioral intervention exposure are generally considered desirable, albeit expensive. Nevertheless, for all of the discussions about intervention dose effects, there have been few intervention studies that have systematically manipulated intervention dosage.

In an unpublished study with men who have sex with men, a comparison was made between interventions of three different lengths while keeping the primary components constant: (1) a full-day skills training workshop; (2) an abbreviated 3-hour skills training workshop; or (3) a brief 2-hour session. All of the interventions contained the same components and activities that varied in duration and all three conditions consisted of small group formats and were delivered in a community setting. The results, however, failed to indicate any differences between conditions, with no positive outcomes from any of the intervention formats. Thus, this particular study was unable to provide information about the value of high and low dose interventions (personal communication, J. A. Kelly, November, 1996).

Determining how much intervention is required for positive change also depends on the targeted outcomes. Increasing knowledge about HIV risks, shifting attitudes toward accepting condoms, increasing intentions to use condoms, increasing condom use, and maintaining condom use during every act of intercourse are all different outcomes that will likely require different types and amounts of intervention. Another related and unresolved issue in the behavioral intervention literature is establishing what constitutes an acceptable outcome from a brief prevention intervention. Videotapes, for example, increase knowledge and change AIDS-related attitudes, but there is no evidence that exposure to video messages alone change risk-related behaviors (Kalichman, 1996). It is therefore questionable as to whether videotapes constitute a behavior change intervention, although they are clearly an effective educational tool. Brief, single-session counseling has also shown limited promise for producing meaningful behavioral changes. From a motivational perspective, however, such brief interventions may play important roles in moving people to a state of readiness to change and potentially enhancing behavioral outcomes of more intensive interventions.

There are two simultaneous and competing demands placed on the amount of time allotted to HIV risk-reduction interventions. On the one hand, longer interventions provide greater exposure and more opportunities to practice new skills; on the other hand, brief interventions are more feasible to conduct and are more likely to be useful in public health settings. The majority of face-to-face HIV risk-reduction interventions in the research literature have been delivered in multiple sessions, usually between four and eight sessions lasting 1 to 2 hours each. Multiple sessions allow interventionists to space out components, use homework assignments to reinforce content, and provide participants with time to self-monitor targeted behaviors. Multiple sessions also afford more opportunities for social supports and social reinforcements for behavior change efforts than do single-session interventions. These potential benefits must be balanced against the burdens placed on participants and organizational resources.

ISSUES IN CONDUCTING
INTERVENTION RESEARCH

The gold standard in prevention research is the randomized controlled trial, where members of a target population are recruited and randomly assigned to receive an experimental intervention or comparison condition, allowing for the observation of differential effects on targeted outcomes. The influence of biomedical research on behavioral HIV prevention studies is most evident in the acceptance of the randomized design as the basis for determining intervention effectiveness. AIDS behavioral research has moved toward adopting a framework that captures the goals of biomedical clinical research. Based on biomedical models, research proceeds in a series of four phases. In Phase I studies, new intervention ideas are identified through exploratory methods that examine the safety of an intervention. Phase II studies are small in scale and test the efficacy of interventions. In Phase III trials, larger studies rigorously test the effectiveness of an intervention in relation to the standard of care or an alternative treatment. Finally, interventions that advance to Phase IV trials are tested for effects on disease-related outcomes in community settings, usually through large multisite efforts. The implications of structuring behavioral prevention research in a framework that was established for biomedical interventions allows for greater latitude on the part of behavioral intervention scientists and funders.

HIV-prevention intervention research faces many challenges. Studies at every phase of a research program must make critical decisions regarding definitions of target populations, imposing study entry criteria, selecting a control or comparison condition, instituting a randomization procedure, and controlling for contamination across conditions.

Defining Target Populations

The content and context of HIV prevention interventions is dependent on the intended audience and where that group is placed in the AIDS epidemic. Prevention interventions will have their greatest impact, and therefore their greatest relevance, when populations with the highest rates of HIV seroprevalence and highest rates of risk behaviors are targeted. Designating a target population must therefore reflect the epidemic in terms of populations at greatest risk. Although designating risk groups emphasizes demographic, socioeconomic, and lifestyle characteristics associated with risk, risk groups per se are now only meaningfully defined in terms of HIV transmission-related behaviors in populations of high HIV seroprevalence. Selecting populations to target in prevention dictates much of the structure and tailoring an HIV risk-reduction intervention will receive.

Participant Recruitment

Recruiting persons into an HIV prevention intervention requires a well-planned marketing strategy that emphasizes gender, developmentally, and culturally relevant themes. In most cases, materials that describe the study opportunity, such as brochures, flyers, and posters, are placed in strategic locations such as STD clinic waiting rooms, bars, clubs, businesses, recreation halls, and social service agencies. Media announcements and advertisements are also common, particularly advertisements placed in local newspapers. Following an initial wave of intervention activities, however, snowball recruitment often becomes the principle means of recruiting. Participant referral can tap an entire social network into a study. On the positive side, saturating a social network of persons at risk can have a significant impact on the spread of HIV in that network. However, restricting recruitment in a given social network can have negative effects on the experimental integrity of a randomized controlled study, particularly creating the potential for cross-contamination of experimental conditions.

Recruitment efforts are therefore most effective when multiple strategies are used to identify minimally overlapping networks of persons in a defined target population. For example, an intervention targeting men of color who have sex with men may recruit using outreach to several gay bars with minority patrons, placing ads in gay newspapers, and distributing brochures in gay/adult bookstores serving minority men. Snowball recruitment in minimally overlapping networks helps protect against cross contamination. In addition, researchers can document the degree to which their sample is interconnected by examining the social networks of participants. For example, participants can be interviewed to determine overlapping relationships in and between study conditions.

Screening Criteria

Inclusion and exclusion criteria define eligibility for entry into intervention research. Criteria used for study entry usually fall along demographic and behavioral characteristics. For example, a study may be restricted to men who self-identify as gay or bisexual, men who report having sex with men regardless of their sexual orientation, women living in inner-city housing developments, or homeless men. Setting demographic entry criteria restricts the sample to assure homogeneity of study participants. Homogeneity is particularly important when intervention activities are tailored to specific gender, ethnic, cultural, and developmental themes. Restricting study entry to certain demographic profiles therefore assures a better fit between the intervention and the characteristics of participants.

In the case of behavioral criteria for study entry, it is most common to enroll participants who report engaging in targeted behaviors. For example, interventions that target reductions in unprotected anal intercourse will have little effect on participants who do not practice this behavior. One study, for example, excluded gay and bisexual men from an HIV prevention intervention because they failed to meet the following risk criteria: having engaged in at least three unprotected sexual intercourse acts (anal and/or oral) with at least one male partner in the previous 3 months (Roffman et al., 1997). More restrictive entry criteria, such as requiring that the individual report more than one sex partner in the past 3 months, will further narrow the number of eligible participants. Determining behavioral criteria for study entry centers around issues of statistical power and budgetary constraints. Although a person who consistently uses condoms during every act of intercourse and persons who are in stable monogamous relationships may benefit from an AIDS prevention intervention, the fact that their baseline behavior is already at levels that define success for the intervention limits the ability of the study to detect meaningful changes. Including such persons at the outset of an intervention reduces statistical power to detect change and therefore increases the costs of accruing an adequate sample size to perform reliable significance tests.

HIV risk reduction studies will usually screen people for their risk for HIV infection using behavioral criteria, such as number of sex partners in a recent time frame, having recently been treated for an STD, or exchanging sex for money or drugs. Given that responding to a screening instrument is usually the first contact between a researcher and a potential participant, there may be a tendency for people to underreport risk criteria, particularly given the personal nature of HIV-relevant behavioral information and the social stigmas attached to many HIV-related risk criteria. Thus, the nature of the social interaction in the screening procedure for identifying persons at risk may result in false negatives. However, because most HIV prevention intervention research involves monetary incentives for participation, people may be motivated to overreport criteria in order to gain entry into the study, resulting in high false positive rates. Thus, methods are needed to minimize error associated with various screening instruments. Murphy, Rotheram–Borus, Srinivasan, Hunt, and Mitnick (1997) showed that formats used for screening instruments can have significant effects on their performance. Typically, persons are asked item-by-item if they have engaged in specific risk behaviors, requiring public admission of engaging in a potentially stigmatizing practice. In a study of STD clinic patients, Murphy et al. altered the format of their screening instrument to provide people with a list or menu of study entry criteria and asked persons to indicate if they had practiced any of the behaviors on the list without indicating which one. This study showed that using a menu format for presenting screening criteria reduced the number of false negatives for screening people into an HIV risk-reduction study.

There is an additional cost associated with screening people into HIV prevention research that should be considered. Biomedical intervention research almost invariably sets criteria for entry into a clinical trial. For example, only people who have HIV infection, specified immunological markers, and health characteristics are offered the opportunity to participate in clinical trials testing the efficacy of new anti-retroviral medications. The concept of entry into such clinical studies is likely acceptable to most people. However, people who wish to participate in an HIV prevention study are, in essence, requesting education and information. When researchers set criteria for who is eligible to receive such information, they face the ethical dilemma of restricting information from people interested in learning about AIDS. Even when an alternative educational experience is made available, incentives for participation are usually withheld, again sending the message that researchers determine who needs and shall receive preventive information. The costs, both in terms of statistical power and resources, of enrolling all persons interested in an intervention study must be balanced against the costs of restricting participation to those who meet study criteria.

Selecting Comparison Conditions

Experimental and quasi-experimental HIV risk-reduction studies compare an intervention under study to an appropriate control group. In efficacy studies, experimental interventions are tested under ideal conditions. Appropriate control groups in such studies are often no treatment conditions, or waiting-list-delayed treatment conditions. Thus, the experimental intervention is tested against nothing to determine its safety and potential for positive outcomes. Efficacy studies require relatively small sample sizes to detect differences between conditions because the magnitude of differences is likely larger when an intervention is compared to nothing. Another variation of a no-treatment control condition is the use of time- and contact-matched comparison condition, but where the intervention content does not include any overlapping prevention information. Examples of non-HIV contact-matched comparison conditions include the use of dietary–nutrition groups or general health information–education. Waitlist and non-HIV contact control groups provide a best-case test for the experimental intervention. However, one problem with both of these options for control groups is the differential experience offered to participants and differential demand they exert on assessment measures. Persons in HIV prevention interventions know that they are expected to report reduced sexual risk behavior and increased condom use at follow-up assessments whereas participants in control groups may wonder why they are being asked so many questions about their sexual behavior after being told that exercise and good eating habits will benefit their health. Thus, studies that compare an HIV prevention intervention to no-treatment, minimal treatment, or nonoverlapping-content contact-control conditions stack the deck in favor of finding positive outcomes on self-reported measures of HIV risk and risk-reducing behaviors.

Effectiveness studies, on the other hand, test interventions under conditions closer to practice settings. Comparison conditions in effectiveness research consist of interventions that either represent a standard of care or an alternative intervention. For example, an effectiveness study of a brief HIV prevention counseling model may use existing counseling practices such as HIV antibody testing and counseling as a comparison condition. Similarly, an effectiveness study of an HIV risk-reduction skills training workshop may use a time-matched HIV information and education workshop that is completely void of any skills training but matched for time dedicated to discussing HIV-related issues. Thus, all participants would receive equal amounts of AIDS-related prevention activities, but without the potential for differential demand characteristics and differential outcome expectancies that come with no-treatment or minimal treatment comparison conditions. In addition, content-matched control groups protect against bias due to differential incentive payments. Effectiveness studies also avoid the negative community relations that can result from only providing individuals selected by the researchers with AIDS prevention information.

Randomization and Levels of Analysis

Experimental control requires an unsystematic assignment of research participants to experimental conditions. In some cases, individuals are randomly assigned to conditions whereas in other cases, groups or entire communities may be randomized to experimental conditions. The appropriate scheme for randomization depends on the level of intervention and the level of outcome analysis, and these factors have a significant impact on sample sizes to perform various statistical analyses. Practical considerations must also be weighed in randomizing participants to experimental conditions in community field research. For example, the Community Demonstration Projects conducted by the CDC assigned communities to treatment conditions but did not make the assignment based on a randomization scheme. Because of differences between cities in existing community resources, communities were assigned to conditions on rational grounds (Corby & Wolitski, 1997). Similarly, small-group intervention studies may randomly assign individuals to groups in blocks, launching sessions as groups in order to avoid the potential loss of participants (Kelly, St. Lawrence, Hood, & Brasfield, 1989; Peterson et al., 1996). Because the intervention in these studies occurs at the group level, groups are the appropriate unit of analysis. However, most studies analyze their data at the individual level, ignoring the potential effects and interactive effects of the group.

The integrity of a randomization scheme cannot be assumed. Typically, researchers compare participants randomized to various conditions on measures collected at preintervention assessments. Variables for which differences are observed at baseline are considered potential confounds and controlled in the statistical analyses of intervention outcomes. However, a breakdown in randomization procedures damages an experimental design in such ways that cannot be corrected by statistical covariates.

The integrity of an experimental design, particularly with respect to statistical power to detect intervention effects, is seriously threatened by the potential for cross-contamination of study conditions. Participants in intervention and control conditions can be closely associated when studies sample from a single targeted recruitment site or when they overuse snowball recruitment procedures, with both cases resulting in a networked sample. Cross contamination occurs when relevant information is diffused across experimental and control conditions. Using separate recruitment sites or intervention settings for exposure to different experimental conditions may prevent cross contamination, but will confound study sites and samples. Furthermore, it does not help if the two sites are treated as the unit of analysis because two or even four sites will not provide sufficient power for the study site to be treated as the unit of analysis (Fishbein, 1996).

Intervention Dropouts and Study Attrition

HIV risk-reduction intervention studies are often plagued by high rates of dropouts from the intervention and significant attrition at follow-up assessments. Intervention dropouts can cause selection bias in the final sample, limiting the external validity of the study. Intervention dropouts are particularly troublesome when losses differ across experimental conditions, suggesting differential biases. Not surprisingly, dropout rates vary in different study protocols. Obviously dropouts are virtually eliminated in single-session or workshop-style interventions. Studies that systematically vary participant burden demonstrate differential attrition. For example, no treatment control conditions may provide less monetary incentives and limited contact between participants and the staff, resulting in greater attrition compared to treatment conditions. Also not surprisingly, interventions delivered in prisons, locked hospital wards of other institutions suffer few lost participants.

With respect to attrition at follow-up assessments, studies that have the least amount of participant loss are those with the shortest follow-up intervals. For example, St. Lawrence, Jefferson, Alleyne, and Brasfield (1995) reported zero attrition in an assessment immediately following their intervention, and Kalichman, Sikkema, Kelly, and Bulto (1995) lost 15% of participants one month following their intervention. In contrast, Valdiserri, Lyter, Leuiton, Callagan, Kingsly, and Rinaldo (1989) reported 50% attrition at a 12-month follow-up.

A significant problem associated with study attrition is that there are no universally agreed on methods for managing lost participants in outcome analyses. Intervention outcomes can be based on those participants who completed all aspects of the study, treating lost assessments as missing data. In these approaches, dropouts can be compared to participants who completed the intervention on relevant measures collected at baseline. A better strategy involves conducting a treatment by attrition analysis on relevant variables collected at baseline. The interaction effect between treatment and attrition provides evidence for differential loss across conditions.

Another alternative method is to analyze data from all participants, including those lost from the study, utilizing a variety of intent-to-treat and data imputation models. Some models essentially replace missing values with estimates derived from existing data. For example, Kelly et al. (1994) used a multiple imputation procedure to replace missing assessments with data from retained participants matched on key demographic characteristics. This method increased the within-subject variability and therefore increased the error term in the analyses, yielding a conservative test of intervention effects. Imputing data can also involve regression models that estimate missing values, as well as other statistical methods for modeling lost data.

The populations that are most relevant to HIV prevention are among the most difficult to reach and therefore retain. Loss of intervention participants occurs when people move, lose access to a telephone, become displaced, or gain employment. Investigations therefore routinely use incentive payments to attract and retain potential participants. Monetary incentives in HIV prevention intervention research have been shown to reduce attrition relative to nonmonetary incentives (Deren, Stephens, Davis, Feucht, & Tortu, 1994).

OUTCOME EVALUATIONS

Despite the fact that the goal of HIV risk-reduction interventions is to prevent HIV infections, incidence rates of HIV infections have not been the endpoint in HIV prevention studies. Low incidence rates of HIV infections in even the highest-risk populations result in low statistical power for detecting change. Biological cofactors of HIV transmission, particularly incidence STDs, are more common outcomes from behavioral interventions. The small to moderate effect sizes observed from existing interventions further limit the use of disease endpoints as intervention outcomes. HIV prevention interventions have used several nondisease-state outcomes, including increased risk-related knowledge, enhanced sensitization to personal risk, motivation to change, self-efficacy for enacting behavioral changes, acquisition of risk-reduction behavioral skills, reductions in unsafe sexual practices, and increased use of condoms. Outcome evaluations have relied most heavily on self-reported behavior and behavior change as their endpoint. The following sections briefly discuss issues of relevance to assessing behavioral outcomes from HIV prevention interventions.

Outcome Variables

Although there are many potential outcomes from any given HIV prevention intervention, only observed changes in HIV transmission behaviors will result in reduced risk for HIV infections. The effectiveness of an HIV prevention intervention is therefore determined by monitoring four behavioral outcome variables: numbers of sexual partners, rates of protected and unprotected occasions of anal and vaginal intercourse, percentage of sex acts during which condoms are used, and recently diagnosed sexually transmitted diseases. In estimating risks, sexual behaviors must also be considered in relationship contexts. For example, unprotected vaginal intercourse is safe in a monogamous relationship with an uninfected partner but not with partners of unknown HIV serostatus. Unlike other health-related behaviors, risks for HIV infection are inherently idiosyncratic. A person who engages in unprotected intercourse only after knowing their partner has tested HIV negative is at much lower risk than a person who uses condoms with a seropositive partner. Merely counting the number of sexual acts in a given time period as an index of intervention effectiveness can, therefore, be misleading. Proportions of safer behaviors relative to unsafe behaviors are also potentially misleading. For example, reporting that 50% of intercourse occasions were protected by condoms tells nothing about the relative magnitude of behaviors; 10 out of 20 protected acts and 100 out of 200 protected acts are both represented by 50%

(Aral & Peterman, 1996). Despite widespread recognition of the subtlies of risk estimates, unprotected sexual activities are generally tallied to index high-risk behaviors without consideration of relationship context or partner serostatus.

Because no single index of risk or risk reduction includes all of the relevant information needed to determine risk, most HIV prevention studies compensate by collecting multiple outcome measures. Further testifying to the limitations of single behaviors as indices of intervention effectiveness, researchers have used various outcome variable composites to estimate HIV risks. For example, Kelly et al. (1989) and St. Lawrence et al. (1995) used a multiplicative index of risk, where the number of unprotected sexual acts was multiplied by the number of sexual partners who participated in those acts. Thus, reporting two unprotected acts with one partner yielded an index score of two, whereas engaging in unprotected sex one time with each of two partners would yield a score of four on the index; double that of the same number of acts with a single partner. Unfortunately, this procedure assumes equal risks across partners and does not take the serostatus of partners into consideration. This index also erroneously assumes a linear relationship between numbers of partners and HIV risk.

Researchers have also used composites of multiple measures to derive risk index scores. For example, Kelly et al. (1997) and Susser et al. (1996) both developed composite behavioral outcome measures in two intervention studies with persistently mentally ill adults. Kelly et al. formulated a weighted composite of sexual risk, where weights were assigned to sexual acts that took into consideration whether or not condoms were used and whether the act occurred with primary or nonprimary sexual partners. Each behavior was weighted on a scale from zero to five, indicating a range of no risk to very high risk. For example, anal intercourse protected by condoms that occurred between monogamous sex partners was considered low risk and weighted zero, whereas acts of unprotected anal intercourse with nonmonogamous partners were weighted five. Similarly, Susser et al. weighted sex acts on the basis of type of behavior, use of protection, and type of partner, composing a scale of discrete risk categories, ranked in order of risk level. In both cases, Kelly et al. and Susser et al. rationally derived the weighting system by expert opinion. However, in both cases only one expert was used to weight behaviors, not allowing for assessing reliability of inter-rater agreement. Unfortunately, no summary risk index has thus far been empirically derived or validated based on actual transmission risks.

Literacy Issues and Comprehension of Study Measures

A serious drawback of self-administered assessment instruments is their reliance on reading ability. This limitation is particularly worthy of concern in HIV prevention research because many relevant populations are of low socioeconomic status. In addition to being expected to read and comprehend instructions and item stems, behavioral assessments require persons to perform mental calculations in order to report frequencies of behaviors in specified time periods. Because low literacy can pose serious barriers to assessing low socioeconomic status populations that are often at highest risk for HIV infection, face-to-face interviews have been used as an alternative assessment administration format. However, face-to-face interviews do not completely resolve literacy problems because individuals must still comprehend instructions and items. Face-to-face interviews are also expensive in that they require one-on-one staff contact. Still, face-to-face interviews provide the greatest opportunities to explain and clarify measures, offering some assurance that persons understand the assessment procedure, instruction set, and intended meaning of items.

Reliability and Validity of Self-Reported Sexual Behavior

Studies generally show that self-reported sexual behavior can be reliably assessed among heterosexual, gay, and bisexual adolescents and adults using survey methods (Catania, Gibson, Marin, Coates, & Greenblatt, 1990; McLaws, Oldenburg, Ross, & Cooper, 1990). For example, in a study of gay and bisexual men, Coates et al. (1986) reported 3-day test–retest reliability coefficients for various sexual practices ranging from .40 to .98, depending on the types and frequencies of behaviors. Studies of heterosexual college students report similar findings with reliability coefficients around .89 (Catania, Gibson, Marin et al., 1990). However, reliability estimates tend to vary with retrospective time periods, with greater stability occurring over briefer intervals (Kauth, St. Lawrence, & Kelly, 1991). In addition, memory for whether an event occurred is more accurate than for frequencies of occurrences, particularly for high-frequency events (Downey, Ryan, Roffman, & Kulich, 1995; Kauth et al., 1991).

Another major limitation of self-reported sexual and drug use behaviors is the potential for persons to deny and lie about these practices (Aral & Peterman, 1996). Brody (1995a), for example, argued that self-reports of sexual behavior, especially socially sanctioned behavior such as anal sex, cannot be trusted, stating that social desirability, demand, and other biases make self-reports unreliable. Brody was quite critical of self-reported behavior measures and believed that biases have led to inflated estimates of risks for vaginal transmission of HIV infection.

Social desirability can also lead to increased reporting of condom use, particularly in intervention research where the demand to report low-risk behavior is high. This potential reporting bias is illustrated in the CDC's community demonstration projects. People were asked if they were carrying a condom with them at the time and many who said yes were unable to produce a condom on request. These assessments were conducted using brief interceptor interviews on the street, suggesting that response bias is even a problem with anonymous assessment procedures. Unfortunately, critics of self-report have not offered alternatives for collecting sexual risk behavior data.

Assessment Administration Format

The most widely used formats for collecting HIV-related sexual history data are self-administered questionnaires and face-to-face interviews. Self-administered surveys afford respondents privacy, which is particularly important when study participants are providing sensitive information about potentially stigmatized or even illegal behaviors. Studies show that increased privacy when responding to sex surveys yields reduced measurement error (Catania, Gibson, Chitwood, & Coates, 1990). As previously noted, a limitation of self-administered questionnaires, however, is their reliance on reading ability and adequate comprehension of item response formats. Because reading ability can pose a barrier to assessing low-income populations, interviews provide a viable alternative administration format.

Structured and standardized interviews can assure that respondents comprehend instructions and items. Face-to-face interviews elicit higher frequencies of self-reported risk behavior than questionnaires and minimize refusal rates (e.g., James, Bignell, & Gillies, 1991). These findings support the validity of face-to-face interview assessments. Nevertheless, face-to-face interviews are limited by potential response biases evoked by the interpersonal context of the interview as well as the potential for interviewer biases (Bradburn & Sudman, 1979). However, studies that compare responses obtained from telephone and face-to-face interviews find few differences between formats despite sociodemographic differences between persons with and without telephones (Analysis of Sexual Behaviour in France, 1992; Nebot et al., 1994). Studies comparing audiotape versus written modes of questionnaire administration also find more similarities than differences between these formats (Boekeloo et al., 1994).

Realizing the limitations of self-administered and face-to-face interview assessment formats, the privacy of self-administered questionnaires and standardized interpersonal instruction have been blended in an innovative assessment method. Using overhead projected facsimiles of instruments where assessors read items aloud and explain instructions to groups of respondents, page-by-page, item-by-item, participants are able to mark responses privately on their own questionnaires. This method has been used with considerable success in HIV prevention research with inner-city, low-income populations (e.g., Carey et al., 1997; Kalichman, Sikkema, Kelly, & Bulto, 1995; Kelly et al., 1994). A variation of this procedure involves using overhead projections to instruct and familiarize persons with measures but allowing them to complete the assessments at their own pace.

Additional innovative methods for collecting self-report risk behavior data include the use of computerized and other automated systems for presenting assessment materials and collecting responses. Automated assessment procedures have the advantages of not requiring face-to-face contact with an assessor, removing barriers such as embarrassment, feedback from facial expressions, and other social influences on responses. Automated assessment procedures can also include audio presentation of instructions and questions, which is particularly important when assessing persons of low literacy. Unfortunately, automated assessment procedures are expensive and may not be feasible.

Reactivity to Measures

Self-reported sexual behaviors can have reactive effects on subsequent behavioral assessments, where people report greater sensitization to their personal risk and intentions to change their risk behaviors simply as a result of completing self-reported sexual risk behavior measures. Reactivity to self-reported health behavior has been observed with measures of smoking, weight reduction, and alcohol use (e.g., McFall, 1970; Webb, Redman, Gibberd, & Sanson–Fisher, 1991). Assessments of sexual behavior have shown less evidence of reactivity, with most effects being small, evaluated among people of high literacy, and assessed over relatively long periods of time (Fujita, Wagner, Perthou, & Pion, 1997; Persky, Strauss, Lief, Miller, & O'Brien, 1981; Reading, 1983). For example, Halpern, Udry, and Suchindran (1994) found that repeated assessments of adolescents did not significantly affect behavior change. However, this study used archival data from four samples of adolescents who completed either one, two, three, or five assessments over 2 years. Thus, participants were not randomly assigned to assessment conditions and short-term reactivity was not tested.

In an experimental test of the potential reactive effects of sexual behavior history assessments on subsequent self-reports relevant to AIDS behavioral research, Kalichman, Kelly, and Stevenson (1997) administered sexual history assessments to low-income women using one of three formats: (1) self-administration; (2) administration assisted by overhead projections of measures explaining items while participants completed their own assessment instruments; or (3) face-to-face interviews. All women completed follow-up assessments 2 weeks later. The study found that measurement reactivity to self-administered questionnaires and face-to-face interviews primed sensitization to personal risk and intentions to change risk behaviors to a greater extent than did the same assessment instruments administered using the overhead-projected assessment described earlier. The results suggest that reactivity is affected by who is in control of the assessment administration. In self-administered and interviewer-administered assessments, the person being assessed is in control of the pace of the administration. Self-paced assessments allow the respondent to control the speed of the assessment, affording greater time to reflect and potentially be affected by one's responses. In contrast, projector-assisted administration is administrator-paced, removing control over the pace of responses from the subject. These findings have implications for intervention research. Using self-administered and face-to-face interview assessment procedures may prime intervention participants and increase their readiness to change. The assessment may therefore be conceptualized as a component of the intervention itself and assessment procedures can be used to prime intervention activities.

Objective Behavioral Measures

HIV prevention interventions may include a wide array of outcome variables, depending on the goals of the intervention and the theoretical variables thought to mediate behavior change. For example, interventions based on skills-building techniques have included behavioral assessments to test for changes in quality of skill performance. For example, Kelly et al. (1989) used a role-play assessment to evaluate gay and bisexual men's sexual assertiveness before and after participating in a skills enhancement intervention. Scenes depicting situations where a sex partner pressures the respondent into unprotected sex were delivered by audiotape, followed by three verbal prompts. Responses to each prompt, which became successively more coercive, were audio-tape recorded. Kelly et al. scored responses for effectiveness using rating scales for effectiveness of responses. Similar procedures for evaluating intervention effects on verbal communication skills have been reported in other HIV prevention studies (Forsyth, Carey, & Fuqua, 1997; Kelly et al., 1994).

Gordon, Forsyth, Weinhardt, and Carey (1995) identified a number of key challenges to using role-play assessment procedures for measuring HIV risk-reduction behavioral skills. First, the development of role plays must stem from elicitation or formative research. The scenarios used in role plays must ring true to the lives of those individuals being assessed. Achieving personal relevance of role-play scenarios, however, must be balanced against developing a standardized protocol of role-play scenes. Role plays must be capable of generating cues for responses with reference to an individual's life but must also be general enough for use across participants.

The following are four examples of scenes used as stimuli in role play assessments. Derived from formative research including focus groups and key informant interviews, these scenes were developed for use with men and women living with HIV infection and continuing to practice unprotected sex (Kalichman, 1998). Interestingly, the scenes were found equally useful with men and women of diverse ethnic backgrounds.

This week has been difficult for you and you want to forget all of your problems for a while. You go out walking and meet up with some people you know. You go off with them and have a drink to relax. Even though you haven't had much to drink, you feel it affecting you. One of your friends introduces you to someone you have seen before and felt attracted to in the past. This person seems to be making it clear that they want to have sex with you. You feel interested.

While out with some friends and having fun, you unexpectedly run into an ex-partner from your past. You had sex with this person many times long before you became HIV positive. They start telling you how much they missed being with you and that they think of you often. Then they say that they are not currently partnered. You are feeling good and the mood seems right for the two you to get together. Because you still like this person and have feelings for them, you are wanting to be with this person.

Imagine that you had been in a relationship with someone who just left you and ended it. You unexpectedly run into an ex-partner from your past who is visiting in town. You had sex with this person many times long before you became HIV positive. After telling you how much they missed being with you and that they think of you often, he/she asks you to come to their hotel room. You are feeling really good and the mood seems right and you want to have sex with this person.

Imagine that you are in a long-term sexual relationship with a person who is HIV negative. The two of you always practice safe sex and have a very satisfying relationship. You feel particularly good about yourself and your life with your partner. One evening your partner tells you that he/she wants to experience an even higher level of closeness with you and wants to have unprotected intercourse, just this one time. You have very strong feelings for this person and the idea of taking your relationship to another level is very appealing to you.

Coding and scoring responses to role play assessments presents an entirely different set of challenges. Coding verbal and even nonverbal responses to role plays requires a reliable and valid objective coding system as well as reliable ratings of performance. Finally, practice effects on role-play assessments are very likely. Thus, using the same role-play scenes in baseline and postintervention assessments can be problematic. However, developing truly parallel forms of role-play scenarios is difficult because the dimensions on which scenes should be matched are unknown. Even with these challenges, role-play skills assessments offer one of the few opportunities to collect behavioral data that go beyond the limitations of self-reported behavior.

Researchers have also reported behavioral assessments of condom-use intentions. Methods allow participants to obtain condoms in a data collection procedure, such as the use of condom coupons or condom credit cards. Condom coupons, for example, can be redeemed with research staff and with the coupons coded for data collection. These measures have been successfully used as an assessment of participant motivation to obtain condoms and as a behavioral index of condom use intentions (Hobfoll, Jackson, Lavin, Britton, & Sheperd, 1994; Kalichman, Kelly, Hunder, Murphy, & Tyler, 1993).

Follow-Up Intervals

Almost all HIV prevention interventions have reported behavioral changes immediately following the intervention or at a postassessment. Many studies also report additional follow-up assessments of behavior change several months after completion of the final intervention session. Because behavioral relapse following interventions is common if not expected, longer-term follow-up assessments are important to determine the longevity of intervention outcomes. Unfortunately, most studies do not report assessments that are delayed long enough to assess maintenance of intervention effects. In one case, Kelly, St. Lawrence, and Brasfield (1991) collected 16-month follow-up assessments from 68 gay and bisexual men who had completed their HIV prevention intervention. They found that 41 (60%) of the men maintained safer sexual practices. Measures taken 16-months earlier, intervention baseline assessments, showed that baseline risk behavior, younger age, and substance use proximal to sexual behavior best predicted high-risk practices at the long-term follow-up. In other examples, Peterson et al. (1996), Roffman et al. (1997) and St. Lawrence et al. (1995) reported intervention outcomes from 12-month follow-ups. Most studies, however, do not provide long-term follow-ups and cannot examine factors that predict risk-behavior relapse. Therefore, information is often unavailable about the durability of behavioral changes resulting from interventions.

Classifying HIV Risk-Reduction Interventions

Understanding the landscape of prevention interventions requires an organizational framework. One useful structure has been offered by Holtgrave, Valdiserri and West (1994), who suggested a taxonomy of HIV prevention interventions summarized in Table 3.1. This scheme categorizes interventions into three domains: traditional public health procedures of disease prevention that include detection, treatment, and contact tracing–partner notification; public health education and counseling, which can be delivered to individuals in one-on-one sessions or through street contacts, to small groups of individuals or through institutions; and health communication, public health education such as media campaigns and social marketing. This scheme therefore focuses on the intervention technology and channels through which information is delivered. However, in each domain interventions can be delivered at different levels. For example, HIV antibody testing counseling, peer counseling, and hotlines deliver different prevention technologies at the level of one-on-one counseling sessions. Similarly, pretest counseling, health education, and marketing efforts can be delivered to small groups; and health education, outreach, and media interventions can all occur at the community level. Thus, an alternative conceptualization of HIV prevention interventions is a grouping of intervention types based on their level of intervention; individual, small group, and community levels. Table 3.2 summarizes a level of intervention conceptualization of HIV prevention.

Prevention delivered at the individual level has the advantage of maximizing intervention potency by exactly matching activities and components to the needs of the individual. Individualization of prevention activities occurs through personal contacts, such as occurs in counseling sessions and telephone hotline calls. Individual level interventions typically include HIV risk-reduction counseling in conjunction with HIV antibody testing, as well as counseling outside of testing contexts. Partner notification and HIV hotlines are also included among individual-level interventions. A second level of intervention can occur in small groups of individuals. In these interventions, persons come together to participate in intervention activities in a collective experience. Finally, community level interventions involve prevention activities where information is disseminated through large groups of people, potentially impacting entire communities or populations. Community-level interventions include outreach efforts, network intervention, media campaigns, and social marketing. In each of these levels of intervention, however, there is variability

TABLE 3.1

Holtgrave et al.'s (1994) Taxonomy of HIV Prevention Interventions

Counseling, Testing, Referral, and Partner Notification

HIV counseling and testing

Clinic-based, community settings, perinatal care, home testing

Referral

Case management, access to treatment, prevention services

Voluntary partner notification

Provider referral, patient referral

Health Education / Risk Reduction

Individual counseling

Peer counselor, nonpeer counselor, skills training

Group counseling

Peer mediated, nonpeer mediated, skills training

Street and community outreach

Street counseling, condom and bleach distribution, syringe access

Institution-based programs

School-based, work site health programs

Community-level interventions/mobilizations

Health Communication / Public Information

Mass media

Print, electronic, broadcast

Small media

Brochures, flyers

Social Marketing

Endorsements and testimonials

Hotlines/clearinghouses

in intensity, exposure duration, and expected outcomes. The following chapters are dedicated to reviewing individual, small group, and community level HIV risk-reduction interventions.

CONCLUSIONS

Expectations of behavioral prevention interventions have changed over the course of the HIV epidemic. Beliefs about what AIDS prevention interventions are capable of achieving have been recalibrated many times to fit the realities posed by AIDS. Interventions designed to educate and raise consciousness have been successful, but reductions in high-risk sexual practices and consistent condom use have been much more difficult to achieve. Efforts to prevent

TABLE 3.2

Levels of Intervention Conceptualization of HIV Behavioral Prevention

Individual Level

    HIV testing and counseling
    Partner notification
    Individualized prevention counseling
    Couples counseling
    Telephone hotlines

Group Level

    Small groups
    Workshops

Community Level

    Social influence models
    School-based programs
    Street and community outreach
    Social marketing
    Media interventions
    Social action and community mobilization

HIV infections were first driven by a sense of urgency and the pressing need to do something, perhaps anything, to stop the growing AIDS crisis. Disseminating information through traditional public health education programs increased risk awareness among potentially at risk populations. However, it was soon recognized that theories used to design interventions for other health behavior problems could inform and potentially improve HIV prevention efforts. There has been a steady shift toward striking a balance between acting with urgency and carefully planning prevention strategies (Ostrow, Kessler, Stover, & Pequegnat, 1993). The remaining chapters review sexual risk-reduction interventions, highlighting advances and limitations of interventions delivered to individuals, small groups, communities, and the transfer of these interventions to prevention practice settings.

4

Individual-Level Interventions

Public health and mental health services are typically delivered to individuals in the privacy of a provider–client relationship. It has been well established that individualized counseling extends well beyond a particular set of techniques. Educators, clinicians, counselors, and therapists bring their own qualities to the counseling session. Interpersonal style, humor, rapport, sensitivity, empathy, and genuineness account for much of the success in behavior change interventions (Krupnick et al., 1996). Paraprofessionals often achieve success that rivals that of professionally trained counselors (Durlak, 1979), highlighting the foundations that are basic to all helping relationships (Brammer, 1973; Egan, 1982).

HIV risk-reduction counseling blends the therapeutic qualities of mental health counseling with the information-disseminating functions of public health education. Individualized HIV prevention counseling embodies both health education and health behavior change strategies in client-centered counseling. This chapter reviews the major models and modalities of individual risk-reduction counseling for persons at risk for HIV infection. The majority of HIV risk-reduction counseling takes place in conjunction with HIV antibody testing, in both pre- and posttest sessions. Models for risk-reduction counseling have also emerged outside of the context of HIV testing, such as through case management, substance abuse treatment, and HIV–AIDS hotlines. The following sections review HIV risk-reduction counseling as it is practiced across these various settings.

HIV ANTIBODY COUNSELING AND TESTING

The 1983 discovery that HIV causes AIDS quickly led to diagnostic testing for antibodies produced by the immune system in response to HIV exposure. Developed in 1984, the HIV antibody test became rapidly available, achieving widespread access by 1985. HIV antibody testing is among the most reliable medical diagnostic tests available, achieving over 99% sensitivity and 99% specificity (Saag, 1992). The availability of an HIV antibody test resulted in federal assistance to state and local health departments, as well as other public health services, to establish a network of publicly funded HIV-testing programs. HIV testing efforts were initially concentrated in blood donor facilities as part of efforts to screen HIV-contaminated blood and blood products from the nation's blood supply. However, because many people were using blood centers to obtain free HIV antibody testing, the blood screening program inadvertently created another problem by attracting at risk persons to use blood donation as a means of accessing free testing. The potential for persons at-risk to seek testing by donating blood led to the advent of HIV testing centers in primary care clinics, STD clinics, and other alternative testing sites. Facilities solely committed to providing HIV antibody testing now conduct hundreds of thousands of voluntary HIV antibody tests in the United States.

Counseling was formally incorporated into HIV-testing procedures in 1987. Emphasizing behavior change as an expected outcome from HIV counseling has made testing the centerpiece of comprehensive HIV-prevention programs. HIV counseling and testing is now the most widely available and the most frequently utilized HIV-prevention service in the world. As many as 40 million HIV tests are performed in the United States each year. More than 25% of adults in the United States have been tested for HIV antibodies, and even greater numbers of persons seeking HIV testing are expected. Although the costs for HIV counseling and testing services are high, most HIV tests are provided by publicly funded agencies, allowing many people to receive testing free or testing at reduced costs. Nevertheless, it is known that the costs of counseling and testing to public funding agencies are offset by the benefits of early detection, health promotion, and the potential cost savings offered by prevention (Holtgrave, Valdiserri, Gerber, & Hinman, 1993).

Persons Who Receive HIV Counseling and Testing Services

The majority of people who seek HIV antibody testing in the United States are at relatively low risk for HIV infection, with 31% of the HIV tests conducted at publicly funded test sites in San Francisco performed on persons testing seronegative for the third time or more (McFarland, Fischer-Ponce, & Katz, 1995). Indeed, people who have high-risk behavioral histories often avoid getting tested because they fear receiving a positive test result and because of stigmas attached to AIDS and HIV-related behaviors. Still others with histories of practicing high-risk behaviors do not identify with groups labeled as high-risk and therefore do not seek testing. For example, nongay-identified men who have sex with men, and women who are unaware of their partners' risk behavior histories are unlikely to seek testing (Cleary et al., 1991). Women confront additional barriers to seeking HIV testing, including the potential harm of notifying abusive sex partners of their HIV serostatus, issues involving pregnancy and children, and double standards placed on women's sexual behavior.

Men and women are most likely to seek HIV counseling and testing when the perceived benefits of knowing their HIV status outweigh the potential costs (Kalichman, Somlai, Adair, & Weir, 1996; Meadows, Catalan, & Gazzard, 1993; Simon, Weber, Ford, Cheng, & Kerndt, 1996; Wilson, Jaccard, Levinson, Minkoff, & Endias, 1996). Earlier in the AIDS epidemic, HIV testing was encouraged less enthusiastically than today because of potential adverse effects of testing seropositive, including social stigmas and discrimination. Although these barriers remain, medical advances have tipped the scales toward making early intervention for people living with HIV–AIDS a realistic benefit for those who know their HIV serostatus. The personal health benefits offered by HIV antibody testing are valuable incentives for many persons to get tested. HIV counseling and testing also offers an opportunity to deliver effective HIV-prevention services at a time when people may be particularly receptive to prevention messages and potentially ready to make behavioral changes. In addition to the health outcomes offered by the medical diagnosis of HIV testing, the prevention goals of HIV counseling and testing include helping individuals assess their risk, initiate behavior change, and maintain behavioral changes.

Repeat Testing and Counseling

People who are tested and learn they are not infected with HIV may initiate changes in their behavior that could protect them from subsequently becoming infected. However, for many people, the preventive benefits of testing serone-gative are not realized, showing little evidence of HIV-risk behavioral changes after learning they do not have HIV. Testing HIV-antibody negative can also lead to a habitual pattern of testing. Studies have shown that a significant number of gay and bisexual men who test HIV seronegative integrate HIV testing into a routine or ritual of getting tested repeatedly. For example, Phillips, Paul, Kegeles, Stall, Hoff et al. (1995) conducted a study in Tucson, Arizona and Portland, Oregon and found that 51% of gay and bisexual men had been tested three or more times, defined as repeatedly tested, and that 15% were tested every 6 months, defined as regularly tested. Men who were repeatedly or regularly tested were more likely to have HIV seropositive sex partners and practice unprotected oral sex. These findings led Phillips et al. to suggest that repeat HIV testing may be partly motivated by ambiguities and confusion surrounding oral sex, concluding:

> The importance of oral sex as a predictor of repeat testing may be due to uncertainty about risk from oral sex. Thus individuals engaging in oral sex may be seeking confirmation from testing that their behavior is not putting them at risk. (pp. 772–773)

Thus, repeat and regular testing would be expected to be more prominent among men who are uncertain about the risks for contracting HIV through oral sex, and therefore, rates of testing may vary as a function of various types of oral sex and other sexual behaviors. However, a study of gay and bisexual men surveyed at a Gay Pride Festival in Atlanta failed to confirm a link between repeat testing and oral sex (Kalichman, Schaper et al., 1997).

Another study of gay and bisexual men in Australia divided repeat testers into two groups - those who got tested after experiencing a risk-related event such as broken or slipped condoms, and those whose testing patterns were time-related, that is, testing at regular intervals (Grunseit, Rodden, Crawford, & Kippax, 1994). Among time-related repeat testers, using testing as a prevention strategy was among the significant predictors of testing frequency. Having casual sex partners and engaging in anal sex were also associated with more frequent testing. Thus, it appears that repeat testing occurs among persons who engage in higher rates of high-risk behaviors. Finally, two studies have found that injection drug users and men who have sex with men are more likely to be repeatedly tested compared to lower risk populations (McCusker, Willis et al., 1996; McFarland et al., 1995), further supporting a link between repeat testing and high-risk behavior histories.

However, not all studies have found that repeat testing is related to patterns of unprotected sexual activities. For example, using a similar definition as Phillips, Paul et al. (1995), Kalichman, Schaper et al. (1997) found that 63% of HIV-seronegative men had been repeatedly tested (tested three or more times) and 45% were tested regularly (tested every 6 months or more often). In this study, repeat testing was associated with knowing people with HIV or AIDS, whereas testing regularly every 6 months or so was associated with younger age and not being in an exclusive sexual relationship. Both repeat and regular testers also held more positive health-related attitudes about testing than nonrepeat and nonregularly tested men. But contrary to other studies, repeat testing was not associated with unprotected anal intercourse or unprotected oral sex. Both repeat and regular testing were, however, related to condom use during anal intercourse as well as having multiple protected anal intercourse partners. Kalichman, Schaper et al. concluded that both repeat testing and higher rates of condom use reflect positive health attitudes, and that repeat testing functions to meet the prevention needs of health-conscious gay and bisexual men. Thus, it is clear that many people use testing and counseling to monitor their HIV antibody status, but the motivations behind repeat and regular testing require further study.

Variations of HIV Counseling and Testing Practices

Guidelines for HIV counseling and testing have been set forth by the Centers for Disease Control and Prevention and similar governmental agencies in other countries with the intent of incorporating counseling into the practices of facilities receiving public funds to provide HIV-testing services. In general, getting tested for HIV infection involves attending pre- and posttest counseling sessions, receiving referrals for additional services, and perhaps scheduling follow-up appointments. Persons who wish to get tested must provide informed consent, demonstrating their understanding of what it means to be tested, an explanation of the different potential test results, and issues of privacy and confidentiality. Confidential HIV counseling and testing parallels other medical diagnostic tests where names and other identifying information about the person being tested are obtained and kept with the person's test results in confidential clinic records.

Information collected as part of confidential testing allows health officials to trace and notify persons who fail to return for results and posttest counseling. Notification is particularly important for persons who are HIV infected. A staggering number of persons tested do not return for posttest counseling and notification of their test results. Many people who fail to return for their test results can be found through confidential records that are available to health officials and others, such as insurance companies and employers. Issues surrounding who has access to HIV testing information is a major concern in confidential HIV testing.

The potential for third parties to review medical records and the stigmas associated with merely being tested for HIV have led to alternatives to confidential HIV testing. In contrast to confidential testing, anonymous HIV counseling and testing does not require disclosure of identifying information to the testing site, assuring complete anonymity. In anonymous testing, persons receive a code number that is linked to their blood specimens. Individuals can receive their test results and posttest counseling when they present their code number back to the testing site. With anonymous testing, an individual's name cannot be reported to health officials and they cannot be traced should they not return for their test results. Anonymous testing is often preferred for the obvious reasons that there are no threats to HIV-test result privacy and individuals who are tested can maintain complete control over access to their testing history and HIV-antibody status. Demonstrating the preference for anonymous testing, residents in states that only offer confidential testing have been known to seek anonymous testing in neighboring states (Meyer, Jones, Garrison, & Dowda, 1994).

Unfortunately, studies have also shown that many persons at high risk for HIV infection do not understand the important differences between confidential and anonymous HIV testing. For example, Kalichman, Somali, Adair, and Weir (1996) found that 47% of men and women surveyed in an STD clinic waiting room believed that a person does not provide their name when tested confidentially. The terms anonymous and confidential may also appear together, as in "anonymous and confidential..." inadvertently suggesting that they are synonymous.

HIV testing occurs in a variety of settings and is performed by a broad spectrum of providers, including primary care physicians, nurses, public health educators, and peer counselors. The reluctance of many at risk individuals to seek testing has led to efforts to bring testing options directly to the person. Thus, in addition to testing in clinics, hospitals, doctors' offices, and outreach services, people are able to get tested in bars, clubs, bathhouses, brothels, shooting galleries, and in their own homes. Substance-use treatment centers, psychiatric hospitals, prisons, and homeless shelters are also among the many service-providing agencies that routinely offer HIV counseling and testing. Regardless of where testing occurs, however counseling is considered an essential element of the HIV testing experience.

Pretest Counseling

Pretest counseling typically occurs in a single session along with and just before collecting blood specimens. Guidelines for pretest counseling are grounded in client-centered approaches, reflecting a blend of mental health services with public health education. Individuals are offered personalized information in a manner intended to serve as feedback on their own unique behavioral history as it pertains to risk for HIV infection. Assuming that such guidelines are followed, counseling is tailored to individual needs, circumstances, resources, and states of readiness to change (Gerber et al., 1993). Counseling begins with a personalized and realistic examination of an individual's behavior and past efforts to change risk behaviors as appropriate for their cultural, developmental, and emotional needs (Doll & Kennedy, 1994). Guidelines for pretest counseling stress establishing a nonjudgmental, genuinely caring relationship with the testing client, at least as best as can be developed in 10 or 15 minutes. Ideally, pretest counseling explores the person's decision to get tested, ensuring that they really want to continue the testing process. The context of pretest counseling involves conducting a comprehensive personal assessment of sexual and drug use behaviors geared toward increasing awareness of actual risks and assuming responsibility for one's own behavior (Gerber et al., 1993). The educational process of pretest counseling can also serve to relieve anxieties that result from beliefs in myths that drive misperceptions of risk. Finally, pretest counseling ideally develops a personalized risk-reduction plan, resulting from the risk assessment and negotiation process between the counselor and client. Risk-reduction planning hinges on setting realistic goals for behavior and lifestyle changes, including identifying specific steps that move the person toward ultimately reducing their risk for HIV infection/transmission. The pretest counseling session is followed by collecting blood specimens and scheduling a return appointment for posttest counseling and notification of test results.

HIV Testing Procedures

As described elsewhere (Kalichman, 1995), the most widely used HIV tests detect antibodies to the virus rather than the presence of HIV itself. Antibodies produced by the immune system provide immunologic evidence for HIV infection. Antibody tests are safer and less expensive to perform than actual viral detection procedures because antibody tests do not require direct contact with HIV (Glasner & Kaslow, 1990; Saag, 1992).

Blood serum is first analyzed through an enzyme-linked immunosorbent assay (ELISA) or enzyme immune assay (EIA) that detects antibodies to HIV. ELISA tests are performed as an initial screening because they are highly sensitive to HIV antibodies. If an ELISA test is negative, antibodies are not detected, and it is highly unlikely that the person is HIV infected; ELISA tests have very low false negative rates. However, positive ELISA tests must be repeated because the procedure lacks specificity to HIV antibodies. Therefore, it is likely that an ELISA result could be a false positive. After a specimen repeatedly tests positive on ELISA, the result is confirmed using a western blot procedure. Like ELISA, western blot detects HIV antibodies, but the western blot technique is highly specific to exact antigens (Saag, 1992). A positive western blot result means detection of two out of three precise antigen groups from components of the virus. This level of specificity substantially reduces the chances for false positive results. Thus, both a positive repeated ELISA screening test and a positive western blot confirmatory test are required for diagnosing HIV infection (Bartlett, 1993).

HIV antibody testing is now among the most accurate diagnostic tools in medicine (Bartlett, 1993; Mortimer, 1988). In tests that indicate a false negative result (i.e., that the person is not found infected when he or she really is infected), the most common cause is that the blood sample was collected during the window period before HIV antibodies developed (Bartlett, 1993; Mortimer, 1988). A person cannot, therefore, know they are HIV infected during the incubation period, although HIV can be transmitted to others during this time. The potential for false negative tests requires that all persons who receive this result get tested again approximately three months later. People who test HIV positive and have no identifiable risk history should also be retested, although false positives only seem to result from laboratory errors (Bartlett, 1993).

In addition to receiving either a positive or negative result, a third possible testing outcome is an indeterminate result; neither conclusively positive nor negative. Indeterminate HIV test results usually occur when the ELISA test is positive, and only one of the two required specific antigens is detected by western blot. Ambiguous results most commonly occur when individuals infected with HIV are in the process of developing antibodies, and requires that the test be repeated 2 to 6 months later.

Posttest Counseling and Partner Notification

The nature of posttest counseling depends on the three possible HIV test results: seronegative, seropositive, or indeterminant. Testing HIV seropositive requires that posttest counseling emphasizes a thorough mental health assessment, including evaluations of suicide potential, coping resources, and available social supports. Referrals to HIV-related medical and social services must also be made at the seropositive posttest counseling session. Issues involved in notifying past sexual or needle sharing partners of their potential risks must also be discussed.

Posttest Counseling. The prevention functions of posttest counseling, such as revisiting the risk-reduction plan formulated in pretest counseling, reinforcing behavioral changes, and problem solving barriers to behavior change should also occur for seropositive persons, but these activities become secondary to the coping and supportive functions of caring for the newly diagnosed person. It must also be noted, however, that people who test HIV seropositive retain little information provided to them during posttest counseling anyway (Grant & Anns, 1988; Perry & Markowitz, 1988; Perry et al. 1993), highlighting the importance of follow-up sessions for people who test seropositive.

Posttest counseling for people who test HIV seronegative focuses on HIV risk-reduction, with a particular emphasis on reviewing the risk-reduction plan formulated at pretest counseling. Posttest counseling offers the opportunity to use problem-solving strategies to address barriers to implementing risk-reduction plans, making adjustments to the risk-reduction plan to facilitate behavior change, and reinforcing attempts to change risk behaviors (Gerber et al., 1993). Role playing risky scenarios may occur in posttest counseling sessions. These activities can help individuals overcome problems in initiating behavior changes, including negotiating condom use, initiating safer sex, and practicing needle hygiene with partners. Referrals to additional prevention services can also be made for seronegative persons, including information about mental health counseling services, substance abuse treatment, and additional prevention education. Finally, people who test HIV seronegative, particularly those with high-risk histories, are recommended to be retested 3 to 6 months later to confirm that their initial HIV test was not conducted during the window period between HIV exposure and seroconversion. In summary, posttest counseling for both persons who test HIV seropositive and seronegative ideally includes risk reducing counseling for behavioral changes, although the emphasis for HIV seropositive persons is placed on strategies for coping with their diagnosis and accessing medical care. Table 4.1 presents a brief description of pre- and posttest counseling sessions.

Partner Notification. Partner notification and contact tracing are traditional public health interventions that include locating and informing past sex and drug-using partners that they may be at risk and can be conducted either by the person who tests seropositive (patient referral), or by health officials (provider referral). Partner notification, originally referred to as contact tracing in STD prevention, is a public health intervention that includes interviewing newly diagnosed person (the index case), identifying potentially exposed partners, and notifying partners of their potential risks for infection. The CDC (1988) described partner notification as follows:

> Partner notification begins with a discussion between the index patient and a trained counselor. This "interview" covers the patient's risk factors, the disease process, its course and complications, and sex partners who may be at risk of infection. Divulging the names of sex partners (and, with HIV, needle-sharing partners) during the interview is always voluntary. Assuring confidentiality—protecting the patient's identity and privacy of named partners—is of paramount importance in securing the cooperation of patients and in successfully carrying out the partner notification process.

> Notifying partners identified though the interview process was performed almost entirely by trained health department professionals until the mid-1970's when health departments adopted new methodologies to carry out partner notification. In most programs, patients are now offered the option of notifying their own sex partners and referring them for assessment and treatment. Having

TABLE 4.1

Structure and Content of CDC Recommendations for Pre- and Post-HIV
Antibody Test Counseling

Pretest Session

Establish the reason for testing	Explore why person has sought testing Discuss sexual and drug use history Conduct a thorough risk assessment Establish the client's reason or goal of testing
Provide information	Explain HIV and AIDS Explain the steps of antibody testing Explain the meaning of positive and negative results Discuss the possibilities of false positive, false negative, and indeterminate test results Explore risk-reduction strategies

Explain implications of testing	Discuss the benefits of testing
	Discuss the risks and alternatives to testing
	Describe and explain confidentiality, reporting, and
	    partner notification Discuss the stress of waiting for
	    results and potential reactions to test results
	Discuss confidential or anonymous testing conditions

Initiate testing procedure	Obtain informed consent for test Explain that results can only be given in person Arrange a return appointment for a face-to-face visit

Posttest Session

Communicate test results	Provide the test result Assess client's understanding of the result Encourage expressions of feelings and reactions
Assess response to results	Assess the client's psychological conditions Develop a plan for overcoming adverse reactions Arrange additional psychological and social services

Discuss consequences
    of results
	Discuss the health and reproductive consequences of
	    result
	Arrange medical follow-up

Risk-reduction counseling	Review the ways that HIV is transmitted Review the client's risk-producing behaviors and how they may be modified Assess the client's commitment to risk reduction Arrange for partner notification when appropriate

*a health department professional inform partners, however, is still preferred by
many patients who wish to remain anonymous. (p. 2)*

Also according to the CDC (1988), partner notification is conducted under
six guiding principles: *Voluntarism*, disclosure of partner names is voluntary
and in no way affects services provided to the index patient; *confidentiality*,
names of partners are secured for field investigation only and the identity of

index patients is concealed; *accessibility*, partner notification should be offered to all HIV-seropositive clients; *quality assurance*, professional conduct is monitored by health department officials; *provide information*, all clients are to be educated regardless of their participation in partner notification; and *target services*, tailoring partner notification to the needs of specific populations.

There are three general models of partner notification: patient, provider, and a combined approach. In patient referral, the index patient agrees to notify partners at risk for exposure. On the up side, patient referral is less expensive and potentially less intrusive than provider notification. On the down side, index patients must reveal their HIV status with the risk of stigma, discrimination, and other adverse reactions. Provider referral notification involves disclosure of partner names to health officials who then notify partners through field visits. On the up side, provider referral can preserve the anonymity of the index client and increases the chances for notification occurring. However, provider referral is costly and can be viewed as an intrusion of the state on personal privacy. In combined approaches, a mixed patient and provider referral occurs when the patient makes some contacts and the health department contacts others. Patients may request that health workers assist them in notifying partners, or may make their own attempt to notify but fall back on providers for assistance. A limited amount of research has suggested that seropositive persons often fail to contact past partners to notify them of their risks (Cates, Toomey, Havlak, Bowen, & Hinman, 1990; Landis, Schoenbach, Weber, Mittal et al., 1992), making patient referral notification less reliable than provider referral. However, it is not surprising that people do not follow through in notifying past sex partners given the many problems in disclosing HIV serostatus even to current sex partners (Marks et al., 1994).

Despite its long history, dating back to syphilis prevention of the 1930s, there is surprisingly little data evaluating the efficacy of partner notification. It is not known how many people refuse to participate in partner notification, what happens during notification, and what positive and negative outcomes result from partner notification. One study found that 87% of partners notified of their risk for HIV exposure believed that being contacted was the right thing and 92% believed that partner notification services should continue (Jones et al., 1990). However, in terms of overall performance, a CDC external review panel concluded that partner notification programs sometimes fail to adhere to CDC standards of professionalism and do not respect the confidentiality of clients. Some partner notification programs were found punitive and counterproductive to effective prevention. These findings led the CDC to revise their partner notification guidelines in 1997.

Partner notification in HIV is complicated by the psychological vulnerability of people at the HIV posttest counseling session. Disclosure of persons' names who are potentially exposed to HIV could involve illegal behaviors, placing partners and index patients at risk. Index patients may also be at risk for abandonment, abuse, and even violence as a result of partner notification (Rothenberg & Paskey, 1995). Thus, similar to other problems that involve a duty to warn, partner notification works best when persons can consider disclosing partner names in advance of being asked to do so (Bayer & Toomey, 1992; Kalichman, 1995). In this regard, there is no substitute for clear and properly informed consent.

Ideals Versus Realities of HIV Testing and Counseling

Unlike the standards developed for HIV antibody detection in laboratory analyses, standards and guidelines for HIV pre- and posttest counseling are difficult to regulate, making standardization and quality control for counseling nearly impossible. HIV counseling is therefore not uniformly delivered across testing sites and varies in individual testing sites depending mostly on the skills and commitment of individual counselors. Research conducted by the Centers for Disease Control and Prevention has evaluated publicly funded counseling and testing sites, showing that counselors rarely develop risk-reduction plans with their clients (Doll & Kennedy, 1994). Instead of following guidelines for client-centered HIV-prevention counseling, many counselors lecture clients about their potential risks and instruct clients to change their behavior. Counseling sessions for people who test HIV seronegative last an average of 10 minutes and 40% of public providers do not provide intervention elements that even resemble the CDC's counseling guidelines. Similar problems in delivering quality HIV counseling services exist in private testing facilities, where only 28% of providers counsel clients. Thus, the potential for HIV counseling and testing practices to impact on risk behavior seems remote.

Another pervasive problem in HIV counseling and testing mentioned earlier is the failure of people to return for their test results, and therefore never receive any posttest counseling. Failure to return for test results and posttest counseling is particularly troublesome for people who are tested anonymously and are in fact HIV infected, rendering them untraceable and unnotifiable. Valdiserri, Lyter, Leviton, Callahan, and Kingsley, (1993) found that about half of people who receive pretest counseling and have their blood collected do not voluntarily return for test results and posttest counseling. Of people who go to clinics or other testing sites specifically to get tested, nearly one in four do not return. The greatest return rates for test results occur among people who are tested in physicians' offices and freestanding testing centers, whereas the lowest return rates occur for STD and family planning clinics. Incomplete counseling and testing, where persons are tested but do not receive their results, therefore represents a high cost with no known preventive benefit.

New HIV Testing Technologies

Technological advances in HIV antibody testing have led to greater access to testing services, but have also created several new challenges, particularly with regard to realizing the potential preventive benefits of counseling associated with clinic-based testing. In Spring of 1996, the U.S. Food and Drug Administration approved the first HIV test delivered entirely outside of a clinical service setting. The first home HIV testing systems were methods for collecting blood specimens, with the immunological assays performed in remote laboratories. Kits for home testing are sold over the counter and although the diagnostic functions of the test are essentially the same as those obtained through clinic-based testing, other aspects of testing are altered to accommodate the home test procedures.

Home testing kits cannot conceivably include pretest counseling. One marketed home testing kit, for example, included an information booklet to explain the facts about HIV and AIDS, describe HIV transmission, discuss HIV prevention, and summarize the legal issues related to testing for HIV (Direct Access, 1996). In home testing, a booklet therefore replaces pretest counseling. Home testing does not typically involve conducting a test at home, but rather the person uses a finger lancet to collect a few drops of blood on blotter paper, which is then placed in a mailer that is returned to a laboratory that performs the test. After waiting as little as 3 days, the person telephones the testing center for notification of their results. Posttest notification for people who test HIV seropositive involves discussing the meaning of the test results over the telephone with a counselor. Thus, people who test HIV seropositive receive posttest counseling in a similar manner as clients who visit a face-to-face counseling and testing center. In contrast, people who test HIV seronegative first receive their test results delivered by an audio-taped telephone message with an option to talk with a counselor.

The absence of pretest counseling, the fact that all posttest counseling occurs by telephone, and that seronegatives do not necessarily receive any counseling has raised questions about the ethics of home HIV testing and counseling, suggesting that such procedures will have limited preventive benefits. Arguments in favor of home HIV testing, however, point out the value of providing greater options from which persons can choose and the value of increased access to testing (Bayer, Stryker, & Smith, 1995). Many people with high-risk behavior histories prefer home testing and may not be willing to get tested through clinic-based services (Phillips, Flatt, Morrison, & Coates, 1995).

Advances in testing technologies will continue to increase testing options and challenge us to rethink counseling procedures in new testing contexts. Rapid tests that allow for collecting blood specimens and receiving test results in a single session, saliva antibody tests, urine tests, and other new technologies have either arrived or are on the horizon (Schopper & Vercauteren, 1996). At-home tests that do not require sending blood specimens to a lab, functioning in the same way as at-home pregnancy tests, are also becoming available. Thus, advances in the development of counseling technologies are quickly being outdated by advances in testing technologies, requiring constant rethinking, revising, and reinventing of counseling in conjunction with HIV-antibody testing.

Continued Sexual Risk Behavior
After Testing HIV Seropositive

Among the greatest disappointments in HIV testing and counseling is its limited effects on the risk behaviors of many persons who test HIV seropositive. Studies of men who have received HIV-seropositive antibody test results indicate that a significant number continue to engage in sexual behaviors that place their sex partners and themselves at considerable risk for transmission of HIV and other sexually transmitted infections (Cleary et al., 1991; Higgins et al., 1991; Lemp et al., 1994). A report from the Multicenter AIDS Cohort Study found that 35% of HIV-seropositive men had engaged in insertive anal intercourse in the previous 6 months (Robins, Dew, Davidson, Penkower, & Becker, 1994), and as many as 40% of HIV-seropositive blood donors may continue high-risk sexual practices following HIV test result notification (Cleary et al., 1991). Similarly, HIV-seropositive men who use injection drugs demonstrate continued risky injection and sexual practices after learning they are HIV infected (Rhodes, Donoghoe, Hunter, & Stimson, 1993). For example, Singh et al. (1993) found that 29% of HIV-seropositive injection drug users continued sexual risk behaviors after receiving their HIV antibody test results. As the number of men who become infected with HIV increases and as persons continue to live with HIV for longer periods of time, there is an increasingly urgent need to develop interventions that support the long-term behavioral changes required of HIV seropositive men.

Research suggests that as many as one third of HIV-seropositive men who have sex with men engage in unprotected anal intercourse, and the rate of risky sex among seropositive men may not be any less than that observed among seronegative men (Kelly et al., 1992; Lemp et al., 1994; Schwarcz et al., 1995; Wenger, Kusseling, Beck, & Shapiro, 1994). One third of HIV-seropositive men attending substance abuse support groups engaged in multiple unprotected sex acts and 34% had two or more sex partners in the previous month (Kalichman, Greenberg, & Abel, 1997). A review of the scientific literature suggests that there are a number of factors that are plausible correlates of continued risk behavior among seropositive men. Studies of continued sexual risk behavior in seropositive men have concentrated on frequencies of high- and low-risk sex acts as well as predictors of sexual risk practices. Identified risk correlates among seropositive men include relationship types, economic conditions, affective states, substance use, and psychological control and behavioral disinhibition. In addition, self-disclosure of HIV serostatus is an important factor in risks posed to sexual partners of seropositive men.

Relationship Status. The relationship contexts in which sexual behaviors occur are an important aspect of understanding continued risky sexual behaviors in HIV-seropositive persons. Sexual behaviors carry different meanings in different types of relationships. For example, HIV-seropositive men who are in exclusive seroconcordant relationships are not at risk for infecting an uninfected partner should they engage in unprotected sexual relations. Seropositive men who are in serodiscordant relationships, however, do risk potentially infecting their partners through unprotected sex. Several studies suggest that unsafe sex is more frequent in primary sexual relationships than in casual relationships (Doll et al., 1990), including serodiscordant relationships (Remien, Carballo–Dieguez, & Wagner, 1995). HIV-infected persons may also negotiate safety in their relationships by selecting seroconcordant sex partners regardless of whether they practice safer sex (Kippax et al., 1993, 1997).

Economic Conditions and Survival Sex. It is likely that a number of HIV-seropositive persons engage in unprotected sex for money, drugs, or to meet other survival needs because the economic conditions that exist before one becomes HIV infected do not improve with seroconversion. Among seropositive men attending substance-use support groups, one study reported that 24% had exchanged sex for money or drugs (Kalichman, Greenberg, & Abel, 1997). A significant number of seropositive men may engage in sexual commerce and survival sex, with 32% of indigent seropositive men surveyed in Atlanta reporting having traded sex for money or drugs (Kalichman, Belcher et al., in press). These patterns could be expected for seropositive women as well, but there are no empirical data available on the sexual behavior of women living with HIV infection.

Negative Affective States and Poor Coping Resources. Negative affective states including depression, anxiety, and hostility correlate with high-risk sexual practices among HIV-seropositive persons (Kennedy et al., 1993). Seropositive men seeking HIV prevention services who continue to practice unprotected anal intercourse are more likely to be depressed than are their HIV-seropositive counterparts who only practice safer sex (Kalichman, Roffman, Picciano, & Bolan, 1997). These findings replicate earlier research that reported an association between unsafe sex and depression in HIV-seropositive men seeking mental health services (Kelly et al., 1993). Seropositive and seronegative men who practice risky sex use fewer behavioral coping strategies in dealing with stress than lower-risk men (Folkman et al., 1992; Robins et al., 1994), and seropositive men who continue to engage in high-risk sex have a lower capacity for coping with sexual risk-producing situations than lower-risk men (Kalichman, Roffman et al., 1997). Depression and coping deficits may precipitate engaging in unprotected sex as is the case for some seronegative men, or depression and poor coping may be consequences of unsafe sexual behavior.

Substance Abuse and Continued Sexual Risk. Alcohol and drug abuse are commonly associated with unprotected sexual behaviors (Davidson et al., 1995). Previous research with HIV serodiscordant couples has found that substance use plays a significant role in failure to use condoms (Kennedy et al., 1993). Seropositive men who continue high-risk sex also report using illicit drugs to help them cope with stressful situations related to being HIV infected (Robins et al., 1994). Research with seropositive men seeking mental health (Kelly et al., 1993) and prevention services (Kalichman, Kelly, & Rompa, 1997) shows that continued sexual risk behavior among seropositive men is often connected to alcohol and other drug use. In prevention-intervention studies, for example, seropositive men who engage in unprotected anal intercourse report greater use of nitrite inhalants than men who only practice safer sex behaviors. In addition, seropositive men who engage in unprotected anal intercourse indicate that their sex partners more frequently use alcohol and nitrite inhalants (Kalichman, Kelly et al., 1997). A majority of HIV-seropositive men in a survey conducted in Atlanta reported past and current use of alcohol and drugs. This investigation reported that 72% of seropositive men recently drank alcohol, 81% recently used cocaine, and 69% reported that their drug of choice was cocaine (Kalichman, Belcher et al., 1997). The prevalence of cocaine abuse among seropositive men and women is particularly noteworthy given the close association between crack cocaine and HIV infection (Eldin et al., 1994). Like seronegative persons, alcohol and drug use was common in the context of sexual relations, with 41% of seropositive men using alcohol and 35% using other drugs before or during unprotected sex. Again, it is expected that similar patterns may occur for HIV-positive women.

Psychological Control and Behavioral Disinhibition
A number of mental health problems have been associated with high risk for HIV infection, including manic episodes, hypersexuality, and serious personality disorders (Kalichman, Carey, & Carey, 1996). Persistent and pervasive thoughts about sex that are linked to strong desires and urges can be indicative of psychosexual disturbances. Sexual preoccupations that encompass cognitive and affective processes characterized by excessive sexual-erotic ideation can lead to excessive sexual acting-out behavior (Barth & Kinder, 1987; Boast & Cold, 1994; Quadland & Shattls, 1987). It is therefore plausible that these same attributes contribute to continued sexual risk behaviors after one tests HIV-seropositive. Research has found that HIV seropositive men participating in support groups and prevention programs who report multiple unprotected sex partners demonstrate greater sexual preoccupation and disinhibition than men with one or no unprotected partners (Kalichman, Greenberg, & Abel, 1997).

Counseling, Testing, and Behavior Change

HIV-antibody counseling and testing aims to reduce HIV risk behavior by determining and informing a person of their HIV serostatus, increasing their risk awareness, and assisting individuals to plan for personal risk-reduction. Research investigating the effectiveness of HIV counseling and testing has yielded mixed results. Cohorts of at-risk gay and bisexual men dating back to 1981, before there was even an HIV-antibody test, showed that significant reductions in unprotected sex occurred before anyone knew the cause of AIDS. Cohort studies continued to track sexual risk behavior before and after the HIV test became available to show that men reduced their high-risk sexual practices regardless of whether they learned their HIV serostatus (McCusker et al., 1988). The effects of HIV counseling and testing have also been examined in rigorous randomized field studies. For example, a study that compared Australian men who received either counseling, testing, or both counseling and testing found that the combination resulted in greater risk-reduction than either counseling or testing alone (Ross, 1988). In a study of men and woman attending U.S. health clinics, patients received educational information in the form of pamphlets, a 15-minute videotape, and then a 10-minute counseling session. After receiving these educational experiences, participants were randomly assigned to either receive HIV-antibody testing or a wait-list control condition. Results showed that the two groups did not differ and neither changed with respect to HIV risk behavior. However, those who were tested increased the number of times that they discussed HIV risk with their sex partners compared to those who were not tested (Wenger, Linn, Epstein, & Shapiro, 1991). These results were subsequently replicated in a study of college students (Wenger et al., 1992). Additional research comparing HIV testing to control conditions has failed to show positive sexual behavior change outcomes with injection drug users (Calsyn, Saxon, Freeman, & Whittaker, 1992).

Studies of women attending health clinics cast further doubt on the effects of counseling and testing practices on HIV risk behaviors. Ickovics, Morril, Beren, Walsh, and Rodin (1994) studied two groups of women receiving outpatient health care: (1) women who were voluntarily tested for HIV; and (2) women attending the same clinics and matched by race and age but who were never tested for HIV. Using a prospective study design, women were assessed at three time points: (1) an initial recruitment and baseline assessment session; (2) 2 weeks later when women received their HIV test results; and (3) again at a 3 month follow-up assessment. Thus, women were not randomly assigned to testing conditions, but rather the study compared natural groups of women who were undergoing HIV testing versus those who had not been tested. The study found that women who were tested for HIV experienced relief from concerns about their risk for contracting the virus, but neither group demonstrated significant changes in sexual risk-related behaviors. Twenty-five percent of the women who received testing increased safer sex practices compared to 16% of women who were not tested. Thus, although tested women may have felt better after having been tested, there was little evidence to suggest that counseling and testing helped reduce their risk for contracting HIV infection. These results again suggest limited preventive benefits from HIV counseling and testing as performed in typical clinical settings.

Research from Africa, Europe, Australia, and Asia, however, offer more optimistic outcomes from counseling and testing, with studies showing risk reduction following HIV testing. Although cross-continental discrepancies in results are unexplained, they could be due to societal and cultural differences, variations in counseling practices, sampling biases, or other methodological differences. In addition, studies from developing countries involve people who may have limited exposure to HIV prevention and a high likelihood of knowing people who have died of AIDS. This combination of circumstances may enhance the effects of even modest interventions such as counseling and testing. In addition, attitudes toward health care providers and adherence to medical recommendations may differ between developing and developed countries. Differences in culture and AIDS-related experiences may therefore prime responses to interventions (Coates et al., 1996).

One noteworthy study found positive effects of HIV antibody testing and counseling among women receiving outpatient health care in Kigali, Rwanda. All study participants were provided with HIV-prevention education in the form of a 35-minute videotape that used a question-and-answer format followed by a group discussion led by health professionals and then provided women with HIV testing (Allen, Serufilira, Bogacets, Van de Perre, & Nsengumuremy, 1992). Although women were the target of the intervention, their male sex partners were invited to participate. The study showed that 22% of the women reported condom use 1 year after testing, compared to 7% before testing, and condom use was more likely for seropositive women (36% of women), than seronegative women (16%). But the most dramatic changes in behavior were observed among women whose sex partners chose to also participate in the study and therefore receive HIV testing. For both women who tested seropositive and those who were seronegative, nearly twice as many women educated and tested with their partners reported greater increased condom use 1 year later compared to women who were tested without a partner. Most notable were the substantial reductions in HIV infections as well as gonorrhea infections observed after testing. Although only 26% of women's partners participated in this study and these couples represent a self-selected subsample, these results suggest that counseling and testing may be an effective HIV prevention strategy for couples in communities with very high HIV-seroprevalence rates and limited exposure to previous interventions. Still, even these promising results are tempered by reports of increased rates of gonorrhea and other STDs among clinic patients who have tested HIV seronegative.

In summary, HIV testing in industrialized countries has not consistently demonstrated changes in risk behaviors. Studies of women, injection drug users, men who have sex with men, and heterosexual men have shown that behavioral changes have occurred over the course of the epidemic, but these changes cannot be linked to HIV-antibody testing (Doll, & Kennedy, 1994; Higgins et al., 1991). That a single counseling session in conjunction with HIV-antibody testing does not lead to sustained behavior change should probably not be surprising. Standard HIV counseling and testing may have more modest benefits, including the dissemination of accurate information, personalization of risk, delivery of test results in a supportive environment, a source for referral, and a place to help individuals cope with their test results (Doll & Kennedy, 1994). But these outcomes may not justify the enormous costs that counseling adds to testing procedures. The cost savings in HIV testing results from preventing new HIV infections. Posttest counseling appears to offer a window of opportunity for delivering effective HIV prevention services, and has led to theoretically driven models of enhanced counseling for use in settings that provide testing services.

Project Respect: Enhanced Counseling for Testing

As a result of the mixed evidence for behavioral effects of standard HIV counseling and testing, the CDC designed a large, multisite study of a community-implemented, enhanced model of HIV counseling for use with testing.

Project Respect was conducted between 1993 and 1996 at STD clinics in five U.S. cities: Baltimore, Denver, Long Beach, Newark, and San Francisco. The study randomly assigned 5,872 men and women who tested HIV seronegative to receive one of three models of HIV posttest counseling: (1) two sessions of HIV information and education that emphasized correct and consistent condom use delivered by a clinician, set forward as the standard of care; (2) two sessions of HIV risk-reduction counseling following the 1993 CDC guidelines for HIV counseling that emphasized client-centered strategies to increase risk perceptions and use specific, practical steps to achieve risk-reduction; or (3) four sessions of enhanced counseling that included steps toward risk-reduction based on theories of behavior change (Kamb et al., 1996). Participants who received pretest counseling and had their blood drawn were randomly assigned to one of these three interventions conditions. The risk-reduction interventions were scripted, manualized, and implemented in standardized protocols. The enhanced counseling intervention included multiple components and its development was guided by theoretical principles of the theory of reasoned action and social cognitive theory. Project Respect contained exercises aimed to challenge risk-promoting beliefs, attitudes, and behavioral intentions, as well as skills-training activities to increase self-efficacy for making effective behavioral changes. The elements of Project Respect's enhanced intervention are outlined in Table 4.2.

Study participants were reassessed at four time points; every 3 months for 1 year. Eighty four percent of participants completed the HIV education sessions and 86% completed the prevention counseling sessions, but significantly less, 71%, completed the enhanced intervention sessions, suggesting differential dropout due to participant burden from a four versus two session intervention (Kamb et al., 1996). Results of the outcome analyses showed that participants in the prevention counseling and enhanced counseling interventions both resulted in changes in HIV-risk behaviors and reduced rates of STDs compared to health education in the standard care condition. However, the enhanced counseling condition resulted in greater increases in condom use for both men and women (Kamb et al., 1996). These findings support the potential benefits gained from intensive counseling in association with HIV testing and are consistent with the lack of positive outcomes observed from minimal counseling, suggesting that client-centered counseling that actually follows CDC guidelines, or more intensive counseling in conjunction with HIV-antibody testing, can lead to reductions in HIV-risk behaviors.

INDIVIDUALIZED HIV PREVENTION COUNSELING

Individualized one-on-one counseling has achieved success in health-related areas as diverse as smoking cessation, cardiovascular risk-reduction, and weight loss. However, little empirical research has tested the effects of individualized HIV risk-reduction counseling conducted independent of HIV-antibody testing. A number of published case reports have, however, suggested

TABLE 4.2
Project Respect Enhanced Intervention Components

Intervention Component	Description
Session #1: at blood collection	Initial session and blood sample collection; 15 minutes
Risk assessment	Elicits client risk behavior history to facilitate self-understanding of risk
Self-perception of risk	Probing questions about behaviors identified in the risk assessment to increase self-awareness of risk
Risk-reduction attempts	Exploration of past attempts to reduce risk and the successes and failures of those attempts
Barriers to risk reduction	Identification of factors that interfere with behavior change and pose difficulties for using condoms
Risk-reduction plan	Develop specific and concrete steps to using condoms or reducing sexual risk for HIV through optional means; The risk-reduction plan is confirmed as being acceptable and realistic and is documented for the client to take with them
Session #2: result notification	Notification and explanation of test results; 44 to 65 minutes
Myths and facts about HIV	Activity designed to classify preventive actions into effective and noneffective categories
HIV risk continuum	Activity designed to classify sexual behaviors along a range of high to low risk for HIV transmission
Challenging condom beliefs	Tailored for whether the person is intending or not intending to use condoms, this activity uses condom beliefs printed on cards that stimulate discussion about the cost and benefits of condom use
Condom skills training	Education about condoms, modeling correct condom use, and allowing for practice in placing condoms with feedback from the counseling
Condom education	Information about types of condoms and lubricants and their effectiveness
Condom persuasion	Role plays of situations for negotiation and asserting condom use with various types of sex partners
Home work assignment	Taking an individual step toward initiating behavior change between sessions
Session #3: follow-up	40 to 75 minutes
Review homework	Problem-solving barriers that were encountered and process the experience of initiating change
Barriers to condom use	Discussion of factors that create problems for condom use and situations where condoms are particularly difficult to use
Bringing up the topic of safer sex with partners	Generating statements that can be used with partners, responding effectively to partner resistance
Homework assignment	Assignment is to take the next step toward behavior change

<u>Session #4: second follow-up</u>	30 to 65 minutes
Review homework assignment	Continue problem-solving barriers to condom use
Community norms	Discussion of social images that promote condoms including movies, celebrities, and friends; pointing out general acceptance of safer sex
Steps to condom use	Activity is used to examine confidence to effectively use condoms
Steps to long-term change	Maintenance plan for condom use tailored to the individual's intentions to use condoms

that one-on-one approaches to HIV risk-reduction counseling may be effective. For example, Kelly (1991) reported a case of an HIV seropositive man who was continuing to engage in unsafe sexual practices and was seen in individual counseling. Kelly described a cognitive and behavioral counseling approach used to assist his client in initiating and maintaining sexual risk behavior changes. Kelly's counseling incorporated a functional behavioral assessment, techniques for manipulating the environment to avoid risk producing situations, methods for examining alternative behaviors, coping with risk producing situations, and reinforcing behavioral changes, all reflecting origins in traditional behavior therapy. The counseling was clearly tailored to the individual needs of the client and addressed issues of specific relevance to being sexually active and HIV seropositive. Peer support groups were included to help the client develop broader social networks and provide social reinforcements for implementing behavioral changes. After eight counseling sessions, Kelly reported successful results, with his client ceasing high-risk sexual practices. Thus, although single case studies do not provide a basis for generalizing findings to broader populations, this and other cases illustrate the potential benefits of individual, one-on-one HIV risk-reduction counseling conducted outside of HIV-antibody testing.

The effects of two HIV risk-reduction counseling interventions were tested in a study with injection drug users enrolled in methadone treatment in Sydney, Australia (Baker, Heather, Wodak, Dixon, & Holt, 1993). The study participants were randomly assigned to one of three experimental treatment conditions: (1) six cognitive behavioral skills training and relapse prevention intervention individual counseling sessions; (2) a single session motivational interview based on Miller's model of motivational enhancement (described in the following section) with a self-help manual; or (3) a no-treatment control condition. Results from this study were unfortunately not encouraging. Behavioral skills training with relapse prevention did not yield significant reductions in high-risk sexual behaviors, although there was evidence for reduced rates of injection-drug-equipment sharing. It should be noted, however, that Baker et al.'s intervention focused heavily on injection drug use, with relatively little attention to sexual risk and sexual risk-reduction. The majority of time was dedicated to developing problem solving, self-talk, and relaxation skills geared toward coping with injection cravings and lapses to injection drug use. This application of behavioral skills training cannot, therefore, be considered a valid test of individualized counseling for sexual risk-reduction.

Another randomized controlled intervention study tested an individualized adaptation of cognitive behavioral skills counseling for women at-risk for HIV infection. Belcher, Kalichman, Topping, Smith, Emshoff, et al. (1997) examined a 2-hour single-session, one-on-one behavioral skills and motivation inducing counseling intervention compared to a time-matched AIDS education counseling session conducted by the same counselors under the same circumstances. Counseling was conducted with women recruited from the community who reported recent high-risk behaviors, with sessions held at a community service agency that provides meals and social services to indigent adults. Women were evaluated at baseline and again at 1-month and 3-month follow-up assessments. The study found that women who participated in the skills-based counseling reported significantly higher rates of condom use during vaginal intercourse and lower rates of unprotected vaginal intercourse at the 3-month follow-up compared to women who received only educational counseling. The study findings were surprising given the brevity of the single-session intervention, and demonstrate great promise for brief HIV risk-reduction counseling sessions conducted in community settings.

MOTIVATIONAL ENHANCEMENT FOR HIV RISK REDUCTION

Among the most carefully tested models of individualized behavior change counseling is motivational enhancement interviewing developed for treating substance abuse (Miller, 1989; Miller & Rollnick, 1991; Miller, Zweben, DiClemente, & Rychtarik, 1992). Motivational interviewing is a style of counseling that is composed of six general elements: (1) feedback on personal risk; (2) emphasis on personal responsibility for behavior change; (3) clear advice to change; (4) providing a menu of alternative change options; (5) counselor expressions of genuine empathy; and (6) facilitating self-efficacy for initiating behavioral changes (Miller & Rollnick, 1991). Usually delivered in a brief counseling format, individuals are provided with nonjudgmental, objective feedback on their behavior in a safe environment for examining whether they wish to initiate change. Options for taking action and opportunities to build a sense of self-efficacy for behavioral change are facilitated in a caring and empathic counseling relationship. Motivational enhancement interviewing begins by providing individuals with nonjudgmental feedback on the potential risks posed by their behavior, empowers persons to make choices about their own behavior change, guides and supports the initiation of change, and suggests specific behavior change strategies that are instructed and practiced using cognitive behavioral skills building techniques (Miller et al., 1992). Motivational interviewing typically occurs in the context of one-on-one counseling sessions with continued phone contacts and periodic check-in sessions. Developed for use with problem drinkers, motivational interviewing has demonstrated robust effects. This brief intervention model has been effective in reducing long-term alcohol use, alcohol-related problems, adverse health consequences of drinking, and has shown similar outcomes with other substance use problems (Miller et al., 1992).

Motivational interviewing is not grounded in a particular theory of behavior change, but is rather built on techniques from humanistic, particularly Rogerian, psychotherapy (Rogers, 1961). Miller et al. (1992) used the transtheoretical, stages of change model to explain movement from one stage in the change process to the next (Prochaska et al., 1992). Motivational interviewing recognizes that persons must be ready to change before risk-reduction counseling can be effectively implemented. Motivational interviewing intends to lead people toward making a commitment to change their behavior. Thus, with respect to HIV risk-reduction, motivational enhancement interviewing provides a safe and comfortable place for clients to examine their own risky practices and explore changing risky sexual and needle-sharing behaviors.

Techniques adopted from motivational interviewing have been studied for effects in HIV risk-reduction counseling with injection drug users (Baker & Dixon, 1991). In a study described earlier, Baker et al. (1993) compared a single-session motivational interview to both an individualized six-session cognitive behavioral skills training intervention and a no-treatment control group. Results did not support the use of the brief motivational intervention, showing that motivational interviewing was no more effective than the no-treatment control condition. It should be noted, however, that participants demonstrated low-risk behaviors at the start of the intervention, most likely due to their current enrollment in methadone treatment, possibly causing a measurement floor effect. In addition, the study reported outcomes using a categorical risk index score with restricted range that may not have been sensitive to behavioral changes.

In another study, Baker, Kochan, Dixon, Wodak and Heather (1994) reported the effects of a brief, 30-minute counseling intervention based on techniques of motivational enhancement interviewing compared to a no-treatment control group. Learning from the problems of using a treated sample in their previous research, Baker et al. (1994) enrolled injection drug users who were not currently undergoing treatment. Participants were randomly assigned to one of two groups and were assessed in a 30-minute evaluation designed to elicit the participant's stage of readiness to change. The intervention followed the individualized risk assessment and consisted of an interactive, nonjudgmental, and objective feedback session regarding the individual's health and welfare. The counselors used therapeutic techniques to express concern about high-risk behaviors, both injection drug use and sexual behaviors. Counselors also promoted optimistic thinking about instituting behavioral changes. Individuals who did express a desire to change during the course of the interview were provided with a booklet that contained behavioral strategies for relapse prevention. This self-help manual was based on cognitive behavioral strategies, including self-monitoring and risk decision-making skills. Results showed that the brief motivational interviewing intervention did not differentially decrease risk behaviors, neither needle use nor sexual practices, compared to the treatment control condition. However, the sample as a whole did reduce their overall risk behaviors, although not in sexual risk behavior when examined as an independent index. It is therefore possible that the risk assessment itself overshadowed the potential differences between groups. Alternatively, changes from baseline to follow-up assessments could be attributed to factors associated with time after enrolling in the project or other unknown reasons. An additional cautionary note about this study is that it lost 40% of its sample prior to the 3-month follow-up and only retained 44% of the original sample at the 6-month follow-up. Thus, the degree to which this research has sufficiently tested the effects of motivational enhancement counseling for HIV risk-reduction is questionable.

More positive results from a brief intervention were reported by Gibson, Wermuth, Lovelle–Drache, Ham, and Sorenson (1989) who found that heroin injectors who were undergoing detoxification responded positively to a brief HIV risk-reduction intervention based on motivational enhancement techniques. This intervention also included counseling sex partners of the intervention participants. The injection drug users were exposed to two counseling sessions and their sex partners attended three sessions. The results showed modest reductions in unprotected sex in couples following the intervention. Although not overwhelming, these findings suggest that motivational interviewing may provide an intervention strategy that merits further research.

PREVENTION CASE MANAGEMENT

Another model for delivering individual HIV risk-reduction counseling is prevention case management. This intervention approach is usually delivered in public health settings such as STD clinics and HIV testing centers. Prevention case management is defined as a one-on-one, intensive client-centered HIV prevention activity with the fundamental goal of promising the adoption of reduced HIV risk behavior by clients with multiple and complex risk-reduction needs. Prevention case management appears best suited for persons whose lives are complicated by multiple, competing stressors such as the seriously mentally ill, homeless persons, substance abusers, and people living in poverty. Prevention case management therefore represents a hybrid of HIV risk-reduction counseling and traditional case management, a marriage of public health and mental health interventions.

In prevention case management, individuals who are identified as at-risk receive a series of follow-up sessions to support long-term behavior change. Prevention case management incorporates repeated contacts with clients and integration of supportive services that occur in traditional models of mental health and social services case management, including case management for people living with HIV. However, in prevention case management the focus is on risk-reduction. Thus, prevention case management does not necessarily deliver a particular type of intervention, but rather forms a system for delivering a variety of counseling and intervention strategies. Empirical research has not yet, however, documented the content, structure, or efficacy of prevention case management.

HIV RISK-REDUCTION COUNSELING
FOR COUPLES

Because HIV transmission occurs in the context of coupled relationships, couples may represent an optimal level for HIV risk-reduction interventions. HIV serodiscordant couples, where one member of the couple is known to be HIV infected and the other is not infected, show marked changes in behaviors to prevent transmission of the virus, but risk behavior does not invariably cease in these relationships (Higgins et al., 1991). Extensive interviews with gay men in HIV serodiscordant couples have revealed numerous reasons for their continued high-risk sexual practices even when one partner is known to be infected with HIV. Love, preservation of intimacy and sexual pleasure, and length of relationships are among the more common reasons why serodiscordant couples continue to practice unsafe sex (Remien, Carballo–Dieguez, & Wagner, 1995). The couple itself can therefore be considered a factor in maintaining high-risk sexual practices (Misovich, Fisher, & Fisher, in press). The influences that partners have on each other's behavior make the couple a natural entry point for intervention.

There have, however, been few studies of couples HIV risk-reduction counseling. As noted earlier, Allen, Serufilira, Bogaerts, Van de Perre, and Nsengumuremy (1992) showed that Rwandan women who were tested and educated along with their male sex partners evidenced dramatic reductions in risk behaviors for HIV and other STDs. In research conducted with heterosexual seroconcordant couples in San Francisco, the effects of 6 monthly 1-hour couples' counseling sessions were examined (Padian, O'Brien, Chang, Glass, & Francis, 1993). Counseling consisted of bringing the couple together for education about HIV transmission, accessing and using condoms, and behavioral decision making that included choosing to either abstain from intercourse or always use condoms. The sessions included role-play scenarios to help both partners build self-esteem, reinforce confidence for changing risk behaviors, and solve problems associated with barriers to behavior change. The study found that the percent of couples that were using condoms during intercourse increased from 49% at the initial assessment to 88% at the follow-up assessment. In addition, 17% of couples reported sexual abstinence at follow-up. However, this study did not include a control condition, cautioning against concluding that the counseling resulted in the observed behavioral changes as opposed to alternative unobserved explanations.

Motivating behavior change in a partnered relationship is only relevant under certain circumstances. Couples who are truly monogamous and seroconcordant–seronegative have no need to practice safer sex, and there is no basis for recommending them to do so. Indeed, forming monogamous relationships could itself be considered a successful risk-reduction strategy. However, the serial nature of relationships and the realities of infidelity and dishonesty suggest the need for negotiating safer sex in coupled relationships. Couples' counseling for HIV risk-reduction must therefore address issues of trust and longevity in the content of the intervention. Assuring that both partners are in fact HIV seronegative and counseling couples about monogamy and exclusivity are essential elements of couples' counseling. However, interventions that target couples can also capitalize on the opportunity to initiate behavioral changes that could generalize to subsequent relationships.

AIDS HOTLINES AND TELEPHONE COUNSELING

AIDS information hotlines are operated by the Centers for Disease Control and Prevention, state health departments, and local community organizations. The National AIDS Hotline, coordinated by the CDC and the American Social Health Association, receives more than 3,000 calls each day, with nearly 9 million calls requesting information between 1987 and 1994 (Scott & Vangsnes, 1995). Local hotlines also receive high volumes of calls from persons requesting a wide range of information. One study analyzed the themes of 7,000 calls received by a Pittsburgh hospital hotline over a 2-month period, finding that issues about HIV transmission and concerns about HIV risk were common (Polinko, Bradley, Molyneaux, & Lukoff, 1995). Additional research, including studies outside of high-HIV incidence areas (Wellman, 1993) and outside of the United States (Banedetti, Zaccarelli, Giuliani, & di Fabio, 1989), have suggested that individuals who call AIDS information hotlines are concerned about their risks for HIV infection and are seeking information about HIV antibody testing and risk-reduction.

Although on the surface most persons call AIDS information hotlines requesting answers to straightforward, factual questions, a deeper level of analysis shows a need for personally relevant answers. For the most part, questions asked about specific HIV-transmission risk-related practices are framed in the context of personal experiences, such as "I had oral sex with a man last night and I wanted to know if I could have been infected?"; "Can I get infected if I have anal sex and I am the one who inserts into my partner?"; and "Can I get AIDS from having oral sex with a prostitute?" These questions are typical of calls made to AIDS information hotlines (Kalichman, 1996; Kalichman & Belcher, 1997). Thus, hotline workers are well positioned to perform brief risk-reduction counseling over the telephone. Hotline workers may probe questions to identify what motivated the call and identify additional services to which the person may be referred. Hotline workers are usually trained to deliver accurate information and dispel myths about AIDS. However, workers are also often trained in basic listening and counseling skills. Hotline workers help callers structure their questions, asking questions, assisting callers to establish priorities about what they need, identifying what motivated the caller to phone the hotline, and manage crisis calls. As included in one hotline training manual, callers are instructed to "figure out what is the main problem or need that prompted the caller to dial our number" (San Francisco AIDS Foundation, 1994, p. 88). Thus, hotline workers function as telephone counselors in dealing with callers' needs, including those related to HIV risk-reduction. However, the extent to which counseling over AIDS hotlines influences HIV risk behavior or any other potential outcomes remain undocumented.

CONCLUSIONS

The great majority of HIV prevention activities are delivered to individuals in the context of one-on-one individualized services. Whether during HIV antibody testing, STD treatment, family planning, or primary medical care visits, individuals may be asked about their risks, informed about condoms and safer sex, and provided with information brochures and pamphlets. Evidence suggests, however, that these contacts, as they have typically occurred, have had limited effects on HIV risk-reducing behaviors. Nevertheless, services delivered at the individual level remain a viable opportunity to deliver intensive HIV risk-reduction interventions. Individualized interventions have rarely included theoretical principles of behavior change, are not usually systematically tested in rigorous studies, and may therefore have effects that remain undocumented.

5

Small Group Interventions

HIV-prevention interventions delivered at the group level bring individuals together to learn about AIDS, discuss safer sex practices, and participate in educational activities. Group interventions typically meet in community settings such as clinics, schools, recreation centers, and community-based organizations. Groups tend to be intensive, involving several hours of face-to-face contact, and facilitate interactions among participants. Groups can meet in single-session workshops or for multiple, consecutive sessions. Groups vary in terms of their goals, participants, and characteristics of facilitators. In some cases, groups are led by trained professional or paraprofessional counselors, whereas other groups are led by peers. Although group-level HIV risk-reduction interventions are diverse with respect to these and other structural features, group interventions do share a number of common elements. In particular, groups emphasize collective experiences, encouraging members to learn vicariously from each other.

This chapter reviews HIV risk-reduction interventions delivered to small groups in community settings, focusing on the three components of HIV risk reduction in small groups: intervention content, context, and group process. This chapter also reviews the outcomes of empirical studies that have tested the effects of group-level interventions. Finally, the chapter concludes with a brief discussion of innovative approaches to small group interventions as well as some of the limitations of HIV risk-reduction groups.

GROUP HIV RISK-REDUCTION INTERVENTIONS

The first face-to-face HIV education programs occurred in groups, including large community forums and smaller group workshops. Conducted by non-governmental community-based organizations, particularly grass-roots organizations of gay men living in AIDS epicenters, the earliest HIV prevention programs had the goals of providing information about the new threat to community and personal health and instructions in ways to prevent infection. The early group interventions used a variety of techniques to raise awareness and motivate men to change their sexual behavior with a particular emphasis on reducing their numbers of sex partners. Gay political activism was at the center of the first wave of group prevention interventions. Workshops were convened for men to learn about the spread of the new disease and share stories of how it was affecting their lives. Under the leadership of AIDS activists such as Michael Callen and Richard Berkowitz, gay men were urged to make health-minded sexual decisions, to practice safe sex, and to take responsibility for protecting themselves and their community (Altman, 1994).

The first well-organized, peer-led HIV prevention workshops were developed in the middle 1980s, just a few years into the AIDS crisis. *STOP AIDS*, for example, was founded in San Francisco in 1985, and was based on an innovative approach to bringing gay men together to learn about AIDS. Based on a model akin to the Tupperware Party, gatherings were held in the homes of volunteers who hosted the peer facilitated groups. The *STOP AIDS* model focuses on the impact that AIDS has on each individual and calls on participants to take action by answering the question: "What will you do to stop AIDS?" (STOP AIDS Project, 1995).

Safe sex workshops also came on the scene in New York City in the early 1980s. Gay Men's Health Crisis was among the first agencies to organize small group education programs that emphasized techniques for eroticizing safer sex practices. Among the earliest of such workshops was *Hot, Horny, and Healthy*, which was also a peer-led program delivered in community settings. Group discussions focused on how AIDS was affecting gay men and how men could maintain sensual and erotic sex lives while remaining safe from the scourge of the new epidemic. These first safer sex workshops blended the dissemination of basic information about sexual transmission risks with personal, expressive, and emotionally cathartic discussions of homophobia, sex roles, relationships, and values. Similar to many contemporary approaches to HIV prevention, including individualized HIV prevention counseling, these early programs blended disease-preventive information with caring for the emotional needs of at-risk persons, joining public health and clinical mental health models.

The goals of educating gay men about AIDS and raising their AIDS consciousness were achieved by reaching thousands of men who participated in workshops and who subsequently shared their learning experiences with friends and sex partners. However, it soon became apparent that a second generation of small group interventions was needed to push programs beyond providing basic facts of AIDS and techniques to eroticize safer sex. The context within which sex occurs became the focus of new intervention models. Specifically, second-generation small group interventions emphasized risks related to the characteristics of partners, situations, and relationships. Again focusing on persons at greatest risk for HIV infection, namely gay and bisexual men and injection drug users and their sex partners, small group interventions incorporated hands-on, practical learning experiences to rehearse risk-reduction behaviors. Direct experience with condoms, identifying situational barriers to behavior change, and role playing communication with sex partners, for example, were geared toward building confidence in one's ability to actually initiate and maintain behavioral changes. Second-generation group-level interventions were therefore built on the AIDS education and awareness activities of first-generation interventions, but with a greater emphasis on relationships, sexual situations, and interpersonal interactions.

Late in the 1980s, HIV prevention also saw the first studies designed to evaluate the potential effects of small group HIV risk-reduction interventions for gay and bisexual men. First tested in gay communities, researchers used models adopted from theories of health behavior change to illuminate the components of HIV risk-reduction interventions. Like second-generation community-based programs, research-based interventions included several hours of face-to-face contact and blended AIDS information, risk sensitization, and experiential learning. The similarities between second-generation community-based prevention programs and theory-based prevention interventions are striking and make it possible to group them together as one class of small group interventions (Kalichman, Belcher, Cherry, & Williams, 1997). The sections that follow examine the content, context, and processes of small group HIV risk-reduction interventions.

DIMENSIONS OF GROUP-LEVEL INTERVENTIONS

Small group HIV risk-reduction interventions are three dimensional, with intervention content embedded in sociocultural contexts tailored to the population, and delivered through group processes (see Fig. 5.1). The first dimension of an intervention is therefore its content, defined as the experiences, activities, and materials through which HIV prevention is delivered. The content of an intervention is generally found in its curriculum, session outlines, manuals, or other documented sources for what actually happens in an intervention. Although there are exceptions, most small group intervention activities represent four major content areas: (1) basic education about AIDS; (2) sensitization to one's personal risks for HIV; (3) instruction in individual actions that can reduce one's risk; and (4) exploring new ways to communicate with one's sex partners.

The second dimension of prevention interventions is the context in which the intervention content is embedded. Contextual features of an intervention include its themes, values, and language used to tailor intervention activities to the lives of its participants. The goals of contextualization are to assure a good fit between the intervention content and the targeted community and to increase the applicability of the intervention to the everyday lives of group members. The third dimension of group-level interventions is the group process itself, where the intervention activities are played out among group members. Group process emerges from the interactions among group members, opportunities for participation, and the interaction between group facilitators and group members. Despite their essential roles in successful

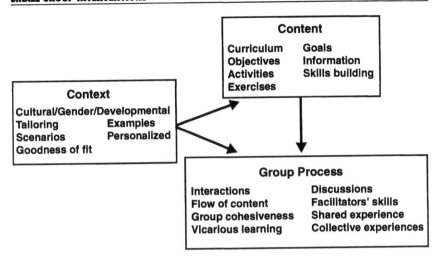

FIG. 5.1. Three dimensions of small group HIV risk-reduction interventions.

interventions, characteristics of context and group process have been less well documented and studied compared to intervention content.

Content

Content analyses of HIV risk-reduction intervention manuals suggest four principal components of intervention content: risk-related information, risk sensitization, behavioral self-management skills building, and communication skills building (Fisher & Fisher, 1992; Kalichman, Belcher, Cherry, & Williams, 1997). Intervention content is easily discerned from manuals and other materials developed to guide the delivery of intervention activities. Kalichman, Belcher, Cherry, and Williams, (1997) conducted a content analysis of curricula from 12 community-based small group programs collected from seven nonprofit AIDS service organizations. Several similarities and points of overlap were found between the components of community-based programs and those of research-based interventions. As shown in Table 5.1, however, not all community-based programs delivered information, behavioral self-management, and communication-skills-building content. Some components, such as basic information about AIDS, were included in only certain interventions. In contrast, time was almost universally committed to discussing interpersonal relationships and role-playing scenarios in which couples negotiated condom use. Thus, the same general template for small group programs is found in both community-based and research-based small group interventions. What follows is a detailed examination of the information, sensitization, and skills-building content in small group interventions, illustrated with excerpts from program curricula and intervention manuals.

TABLE 5.1
Content Analysis of Community-Based Small Group Workshops
for Gay and Bisexual Men

Program	HIV/AIDS Education	Behavioral Skills	Communication	Lifestyle/ Relationships
Stop AIDS SF	X	X	X	X
Life Guard, LA Gay & Lesbian Center	X		X	X
SWIM-II, San Diego AIDS Foundation	X		X	X
Slipping & Sliding, Dallas AIDS Foundation			X	X
Slipping & Sliding, AID Atlanta	X		X	X
Keep It Up!, GMHC		X	X	X
The Dating Game, Stop AIDS Chicago			X	X
Eroticizing Safer Sex, Stop AIDS Chicago		X	X	X

HIV Prevention Information: Just the Facts.   Group-level AIDS education activities provide basic information about HIV transmission, manifestation of illness, and transmission prevention. Risk education includes facts about viral transmission, local prevalence of HIV and AIDS, clarification of misconceptions, dispelling AIDS myths, and descriptions of HIV antibody testing. Group discussions couch information in personal life situations, relationships, risk behaviors, and motivations to reduce risk. Although HIV prevention information may be delivered in lectures directed from group facilitators to participants, didactic instruction is rare in effective small group interventions. Basic information is more often delivered through videotapes, group activities, and games designed to capture the attention of participants.

The content of HIV risk-reduction intervention curricula and program manuals can help identify key elements of HIV/AIDS education. Many interventions have used activities or games to deliver basic information about AIDS. For example, Kelly, Sikkema, and Kelly's (1995) intervention for inner-city women used handouts, lectures and group discussions to educate women about the myths and facts of AIDS. Using myths and facts printed on opposite sides of flash cards, women were prompted to discuss AIDS misconceptions and realities. The facilitator's manual developed for Sikkema and Kelly's (1995) intervention described this activity as follows:

> Let's talk about things you may have heard about HIV and AIDS. There are a lot of myths about how HIV/AIDS is spread. Sometimes there is a fine line between a fact and a myth. I have some cards here with statements written on them. These are things that you may have heard about HIV and AIDS that may or may not be true, and we're going to discuss them. I'd like to ask for volunteers to read the cards. (p. 19)

After reading each card, a group discussion was held to determine whether each statement was a myth or fact. Similar activities have used handouts, posters, and videos to stimulate discussions about the facts of AIDS. Using alternative formats for delivering AIDS education is intended to avoid a classroom-like atmosphere as well as to stimulate participant interest.

Another example of an AIDS education activity was described by Kalichman, Rompa, and Coley (1996) who used a risk continuum to educate minority women about safe, safer, and risky sexual behaviors. Participants were given cards with various sexual acts printed on each, such as "vaginal intercourse without a condom, for the woman," "kissing," and "risk for giving oral sex to woman." Each card had Velcro adhered on its back. Participants were instructed to put each card on a large banner labeled "risk continuum" that was mounted on a wall. The risk continuum was anchored with "very low risk" at one end and "very high risk" at the other end. Participants placed behaviors on the continuum where they believed they should occur on the spectrum of risk. Group members discussed the placement of each behavior, with a focus on exploring how high-risk behaviors could be made safer and with the facilitators assuring that unprotected vaginal and anal sex were always placed under the highest-risk category. A similar risk-continuum activity was included in Jemmott, Jemmott, & McCaffree's (1994) intervention for minority youth.

Research-based interventions have invariably included basic HIV risk information in their content, primarily because risk knowledge is emphasized in traditional public health and in most theories of health behavior change. Thus, Kelly and St. Lawrence (1990) dedicated three sessions to AIDS risk education, describing their educational component as follows:

> *Three sessions presented detailed information about AIDS, HIV infection, epidemiology, and methods of transmission. High-risk behaviors and risk-reduction changes were discussed in detail, including rationale for understanding why particular behaviors posed risk. Whenever possible, local HIV prevalence data was presented to increase salience for the need to make behavior changes. Myths and misconceptions concerning AIDS, HIV infection, and risk-reduction were also discussed. (p. 16)*

Similarly, Peterson et al. (1996), in their intervention for African-American men who have sex with men, included a component covering AIDS knowledge, sexual transmission and drug use, and incorporated a safer sex quiz as well as a large group discussion of common misconceptions about AIDS. In contrast, community-based interventions targeting men who have sex with men often dropped information about HIV and AIDS out of their interventions. The likelihood that gay and bisexual men have been exposed to HIV risk information is high and they may be turned off by repetitious AIDS education. Interventions designed for other populations that have not been as inundated with AIDS education will likely include basic facts about AIDS. This observation speaks to how intervention content changes for various populations, depending on their history of exposure to HIV prevention.

Interventions have used a variety of techniques to make learning about AIDS fun. An example of a game developed for providing basic risk information is found in Jemmott et al.'s (1994) intervention *Be Proud, Be Responsible* designed for African-American adolescents. AIDS education was placed in the context of a basketball game played by dividing the group into two teams, with members rotating answering questions about AIDS, scoring points for correct responses. Using basketball as a vehicle for delivering educational messages illustrates how intervention components are tailored to match the interests of target populations. Jemmott et al. also provided a good example of how open discussions can be incorporated into educational activities. Jemmott et al. used AIDS basketball to describe the difference between HIV and AIDS and to explain how the human immune system functions, how HIV disrupts immune processes, and the ways in which HIV is transmitted through blood, semen, vaginal secretions, and breast milk.

Videotapes are another way to deliver HIV risk-reduction information to small groups, where videos are used to engage participants while simultaneously providing basic education. Brief information videos have been shown to increase knowledge about AIDS across diverse populations (Kalichman, 1996), and several small group interventions have incorporated videos into their educational components (e.g., Kalichman, Rompa, & Coley, 1996; Kelly et al., 1994; Peterson et al., 1996). Small group interventions have also used HIV risk information as a means of encouraging individuals to assess their own behavioral risk histories and initiate discussions of individual life-situations that have placed them at risk. Thus, once individuals know what causes risk for HIV transmission, they are able to examine their own behavior in the context of potential risks.

Risk-Sensitization: Personalizing the Facts to Motivate Behavior Change.

Motivation to change behavior requires both awareness of a threat, usually provided by basic education, and a linkage between risk knowledge and one's own behavior and life circumstances. Kelly, Kalichman et al. (1996) and Kalichman, Rompa, and Coley (1996) used a personal risk continuum to build a bridge between risk information and personal risk sensitization. After participating in group exercises to identify levels of risk posed by various sexual acts, group participants were asked to think of their own behavior and were given a handout representing their own personal risk continuum. Figure 5.2 shows the personal risk continuum handout used in Kalichman et al.'s intervention. Participants wrote their own recent behaviors along the risk continuum as a means of gauging their own risk. This exercise was followed by having participants create their ideal personal risk continuum, showing the safer behaviors that they wanted to try to practice to reduce their risk for HIV infection. Thus, the risk awareness gained through education was used to induce participants to reflect on their own personal risk and set goals for risk-reduction behavioral changes.

Jemmott et al. (1994) included several activities aimed to increase adolescents' sense of personal vulnerability to AIDS. First, group facilitators quoted statistics to heighten participant anxiety about the realities of AIDS, such as:

Every 10 seconds someone gets an STD and HIV can be passed on the same way as STDs; one in 50 people who go to an STD clinic are HIV positive; HIV is

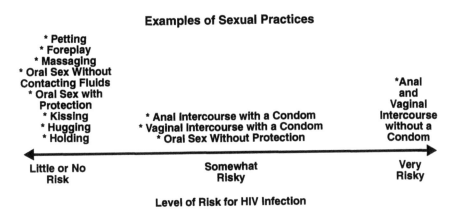

Examples of Sexual Practices

* Petting * Foreplay * Massaging * Oral Sex Without Contacting Fluids * Oral Sex with Protection * Kissing * Hugging * Holding	 * Anal Intercourse with a Condom * Vaginal Intercourse with a Condom * Oral Sex Without Protection	*Anal and Vaginal Intercourse without a Condom
Little or No Risk	Somewhat Risky	Very Risky

Level of Risk for HIV Infection

FIG. 5.2. Example of the risk continuum handout used by Kalichman, Rompa, and Coley (1996).

infecting more people in the inner cities than in other areas; and more teens are getting infected with HIV now than ever. (p. 45)

Risk sensitization also occurred in Jemmott, Jemmott, and Fong's (1992) intervention through the use of videotapes prompting discussions about personal risks. Videos that portray people living with HIV who share common characteristics with the intended audience may reduce the perception that "AIDS doesn't happen to people like me." Videotapes portraying people living with HIV telling their stories and sending prevention-related messages have been widely disseminated for specific populations. Other intervention models have invited guest speakers to deliver live presentations or lead group discussions about how they might have avoided becoming infected, advising participants not to let AIDS happen to them (O'Hara, Messick, Fitchner, & Parris, 1996).

Although general examples of how HIV has affected individuals and communities may instill a sense of personal susceptibility to AIDS and motivate behavior change, such messages may also lack direct relevance to the lives of a targeted audience. Presenting feedback to participants on their own behavior has been used a strategy for linking one's personal history to risk for HIV infection. Two small group HIV risk-reduction interventions have adapted behavioral feedback exercises from *Motivational Enhancement Interviewing* (Miller et al., 1992), a well-developed and empirically tested brief treatment for alcoholism. Carey et al. (1997) and Kalichman and Cherry (1997) extracted information collected in baseline assessments to provide each participant with a personalized behavioral feedback form. As shown in Fig. 5.3, information obtained from a preintervention questionnaire about the individual's personal risk behavior history was recorded. The feedback form summarized self-reported behavior, giving an objective, nonjudgmental look at one's behavior in the context of the HIV-risk information presented at an earlier point in the intervention. Participants were given the feedback form to review on their own, with group facilitators providing instruction in how to use the form. Participants therefore observed how their own recent behavior related to risks for HIV infection and other STDs. Personalized feedback was intended to connect the factual information about HIV transmission with the individual behavior of participants.

Despite the universal inclusion of motivation inducing activities in prevention groups, the field is lacking a coherent definition motivation for HIV risk-reduction. In some cases, motivation reflects instilling a sense of vulnerability through fear, supposedly to invoke avoidance of risk. On the other hand, motivation is at times equated with intentions to change behavior. Still, others describe motivation as a state of readiness to change. Despite the lack of conceptual clarity defining motivation, HIV risk-reduction interventions state that motivation is an essential precursor to behavior change and provide many avenues to enhancing motivation.

Behavioral Skills and Behavior Modification: Self-Regulating Risk-Reduction.

HIV risk-reduction behavioral self-management skills encompass those things that an individual can do to reduce their risk for HIV infection with minimal involvement of their sexual partners. In behavioral-skills training groups, members are instructed in techniques for examining their risk behaviors, their risk producing situations, and actions that they can perform to reduce their risk. Cognitive–behavioral skills training generally includes three fundamental steps. First, individuals are exposed to an example or model, demonstrating a successful execution of the skill. Modeling can be performed by group facilitators or through video presentations. Following exposure to the modeled behavior, the group discusses and often critiques the model's performance. Modeling and discussion are followed by the third step, giving group participants the opportunity to rehearse the new behavior in session. Practice can take place in dyads, breakout groups, or in the larger group usually in the form of a role play. Practice is followed by feedback on performance, again in group discussions, reinforcing performance and providing corrective suggestions for improvement. Individuals in the group therefore take turns practicing and receiving feedback.

Although research has not investigated the independent effects of modeling, practice, and feedback in HIV risk-reduction behavioral skills training, the behavior therapy literature suggests that the full model may not be necessary for skills acquisition. For example, feedback on performance may not offer additional benefit over and above behavioral rehearsal in assertiveness skills training (Melnick & Stocker, 1977). However, there does appear to be an additive effect of modeling and practice. McGuire and Thelen (1983) found that exposure to a model combined with the opportunity to practice assertive communication was more effective than either modeling or rehearsal alone. These findings speak to the potential robustness of the skills-training paradigm. Skills-training principles have been applied in HIV prevention through goal setting, identifying and managing risky situations, cognitive restructuring, and developing safer sex behaviors.

CONFIDENTIAL
Personalized Feedback Form

In last week's survey, you answered questions about your behavior that could put you at risk for AIDS. Here is what you said compared to a survey of 200 other men in Atlanta. You can use this feedback to better understand your risk for AIDS.

Sexual Behavior

You said that you used condoms _____% of the time; the average man in our survey said that he used condoms 30% of the time.

You said that you had vaginal sexual intercourse without a condom about _____ times in the past 3 months; the average man in our survey said 12 times.

You said that you did/did not use a condom the last time you had sex.

Sexual Partners

You said that you had _____ sexual partners in the past 3 months; the average man in our survey said that he had 1 sexual partners in the past 3 months.

Other Risk Factors

You said you had experienced the following:

1. Had a sexually transmitted disease

2. Had sex with a prostitute

3. Had a male sex partner

4. Shared needles to shoot drugs

5. Had sex with someone who shoots drugs

6. Used alcohol or drugs before sex

You rated your own risk for getting AIDS as:

NO RISK AT ALL	SOMEWHAT	GOOD DEAL	EXTREMELY
AT RISK	AT RISK	AT RISK	AT RISK

FIG. 5.3. Example of the Personal Behavior Feedback Form used by Kalichman and Cherry (1997).

Goal Setting.   HIV risk-reduction behavioral skills training emphasizes an individual's capacity to predict and control potentially risky situations. Goal setting is a key aspect of the future-oriented perspective that characterizes cognitive behavioral approaches. Goal setting has been an important element of behavioral interventions for weight loss (Baron & Watters, 1981; Dubbert & Wilson, 1984) and smoking cessation (Borrelli & Mermelstein, 1994). Articulating and strategizing personal goals is a core component of several HIV-risk behavior-change interventions. However, HIV risk-reduction interventions have not used a standard approach to goal setting activities. For example, the NIMH Cooperative Agreement Intervention (Project Light, NIMH, 1996), described its goal setting exercise as follows:

> In order to protect ourselves, we need to plan to be healthy. This group is about protecting ourselves and others from HIV ... We often set goals in everyday life. Goals involve plans to do something. For example, when you got up this morning, you set or had previously set the goal of coming to this group ... At the end of each group, you decide how you want to stay healthy over the next few days and we will set personal goals. Personal goals are realistic, clear, and not too easy or too hard. Personal goals also have a clear endpoint. ... Remember that working toward these goals is hard work. When you work hard to reach a goal, take a few minutes to congratulate yourself and do something special to reward yourself for working on or achieving your goal. (Module 2, p. 10)

Short-term goals were distinguished from long-term goals, and the steps to attaining personal goals were outlined using examples generated by the group. Goals included any safer sex outcome, such as reducing numbers of partners, consistently using condoms, or abstaining from anal or vaginal intercourse. Progress toward achieving one's personal goals was explored in group discussions held in subsequent sessions. Methods for self-monitoring progress beyond the intervention sessions are also useful in tracking progress and goal achievement. Exercises for prioritizing goals, problem-solving barriers to achieving goals, and learning self-reinforcement techniques for rewarding incremental successes can all be incorporated into goal setting activities.

Identifying and Managing Risky Situations.

In many interventions, participants are instructed in methods for identifying environmental and cognitive–affective antecedents that serve as cues or triggers for high-risk situations, including mood states, substance use, characteristics of settings, and sexual partners. Building skills for identifying risk-related cures is often couched in activities that guide people to examine personal risk-producing situations. For example, Kelly et al. (1996) defined risk-related triggers as follows:

> Our actions have a cause, or a reason; they do not just happen. If we were to take the time and examine some of our sexual activities we might be surprised to see specific events guide us into sexual decisions. These events are triggers. Triggers are influences on decisions and behaviors. If we become aware of what they are, then we can be in greater control. When we are in control we can better choose behaviors that we will feel comfortable with. Some triggers that could be associated with sexual decisions might include several possibilities. ... Things that can happen well before a risky situation ... triggers fall into categories, including characteristics of your partner, things about the setting, alcohol, drugs, and other aspects of the situation. (p.16)

In this intervention, the group brainstormed what triggers were most important and were given a trigger identification handout that they used to record at least three triggers recalled from their own risky situations. This exercise was used to raise personal consciousness that led to focused discussions of how triggers can be managed ahead of time and how problem-solving skills can be used to handle risk-related triggers. Similar activities have been included in other interventions, although the exact label for risky situations may differ. For example, in their intervention for African-American men who have sex with men, Peterson et al. (1996) discussed hurdles to practicing safer sex, which included going to bars, drinking too much, and feeling lonely. Thus, Peterson et al.'s hurdles are similar to Kelly et al.'s (1996) triggers.

Risk identification and management was also included in some community-based small group programs. For example, GMHC's program Keep It Up! discussed risk situations rather than risk behaviors, focusing on trigger identification and self-management (Miller, 1995). Group members identified personal risky situations and identified triggers to unsafe sex. The intervention manual stated that unsafe sex happens in specific situations that may involve drinking, using drugs, partner's HIV serostatus, and depression. The group facilitators compiled lists of triggers for various risky situations and barriers encountered to consistently practicing safer sex. Similar to activities included in research-based interventions, strategies and behavioral alternatives were generated by the group for managing triggers and overcoming barriers.

Across interventions, strategies for avoiding or managing high-risk situations were discussed in the group, and individuals generated their own risk-avoidance behaviors. Coping strategies for high-risk situations have included performing safer sex acts, redirecting sexual activities toward safer-sex alternatives, carrying condoms, and avoiding sex after substance use. Identification of risk triggers and barriers to risk-reduction, such as substance use and access to condoms, were also placed in the context of a problem-solving scheme. Interventions have used a variety of approaches to problem solving, but they usually include stepwise planning, thinking ahead, and generating realistic alternatives to avoid or reduce risk. Using problem-solving skills paradigms established in behavior therapy (D'Zurilla & Goldfried, 1971), alternative responses to environmental triggers and surpassing barriers to behavior change may be identified through brainstorming exercises, articulating specific action steps, and clarifying the distinction between effective and ineffective strategies. Techniques such as role play, critical thinking exercises, disputing beliefs, and generating alternative outcomes can be used to explore viable strategies for risk avoidance or risk-reduction.

Similar to goal setting, risk identification and risk management hinges on strategic planning and projecting into the future. Believing that one can recognize a potentially risky situation ahead of time and take action to alter the course of future events leads to a sense of internal control. Thus, persons who lack a sense of the future, those who are fatalistic, and those who lack a sense of controlling their own destiny may not be well suited for goal-setting exercises and perhaps other aspects of skills-training interventions.

Cognitive Restructuring. Cognitive restructuring is another HIV risk-reduction technique adapted from traditional behavior therapy. In the HIV-prevention context, cognitive restructuring aides in coping with risky situations. Techniques such as self-generated statements, or self-talk, to guide behavior toward lower-risk sexual alternatives are a common strategy in behavioral skills training in small group interventions. Rotheram–Borus, Koopman, and Haignere (1991), for example, included self-talk in their intervention for runaway adolescents. To introduce the self-talk exercise, participants were posed with the notion that "if you could slow down your thoughts, you would see that you talk to yourself all the time" (p. 634). Several examples illustrated how self-talk can help avoid problem situations and cope with challenges. After introducing the idea of self-talk and following several examples described in the group, sexual situations were introduced and participants practiced using self-talk to avoid sexual risk situations. Scenarios were presented to participants who were instructed in generating their own self-statements in their own words. The following is an example of one of several situations used by Rotheram-Borus et al. to generate self-statements:

> All week long, you have been looking forward to tonight. You plan to have red hot sex with this new partner of yours. You get so turned on with your new partner that you almost go out of your loving mind. You want turned on sex, but you also want to practice safer sex. You are afraid that you'll get so carried away you won't care about using protection at the last moment. What self-talk would you use to prepare yourself tonight?

Self-talk can be used for instructing oneself in taking steps to practice a new behavior, reminding oneself why a new behavior is important, and reassuring oneself that he or she can perform the behavior. Self-talk therefore serves to enhance self-efficacy for performing a specific behavior and for self-reinforcement following efforts to reduce risk.

Another cognitive restructuring strategy stems from formulating a behavioral commitment or contract to practice safer sex. Behavioral contracts are included in many cognitive–behavioral interventions outside of HIV risk-reduction. A commitment to oneself to reduce risk sets a new personal standard and expectations for one's own behavior. An example of a behavioral contract is provided by the Safer Sex Commitment Contract included in the program *Slipping and Sliding Dallas*. Individuals set a goal for their own safer sex practices and contract with themselves and peers to work toward achieving their personal goals.

Safer Sex Skills Training. Behavioral interventions to reduce HIV risk build skills for initiating and maintaining safer sexual practices. One key feature of safer-sex skills building is instruction in the proper use of condoms. Instructing individuals in condom use goes beyond providing information in a traditional public health sense by including practical in-session rehearsal of putting condoms on anatomical penis models. According to theories of behavior and behavior change, instruction, modeling, practice, and guided feedback on personal performance serve to enhance self-confidence and self-efficacy in one's ability to properly use condoms. Hands-on practice with condoms using penis models may also desensitize individuals to handling and manipulating condoms. Rehearsing condom use in the group setting capitalizes on peer relations to address perceived social norms related to condoms. Breaking down social barriers to condom use can in turn challenge individuals to reconsider their negative condom attitudes. The potential benefits of changing social norms and individual attitudes toward condoms add to the explicit goals of increasing proficiency in proper condom application.

Skills training exercises include demonstrations of the correct placement of condoms on anatomical models, allowing individuals to practice placing condoms on models, and giving feedback on individual performance. Practice is of theoretical importance to building competence in technical skills for condom use, and is important for enhancing self-efficacy for using condoms in particularly difficult situations. Simply practicing condom use may result in positive effects given the research that shows an association between greater experience with condoms and reduced rates of condom failure (Albert et al., 1995).

Skills building, however, will do little if people are resistant to actually using condoms. Thus, interventions often include group activities and exercises designed to directly address barriers to condom use. In some cases, condom skills training is blended into broader group activities to increase its appeal. For example, Susser, Valencia, and Torres' (1994) behavioral intervention for homeless men with chronic mental illness placed condom practice in the context of a contest to determine who could correctly place a condom on a penis model the fastest. Focusing primarily on situations where sex is exchanged for drugs or money, men were trained how to put a condom on quickly and then practiced in competition against each other. Treating condom use as a game in the practice session was also thought to increase the attention and interest of men and therefore served to contextualize the activity to that particular population.

Activities in addition to skills-building exercises serve to increase attention and remove barriers to using condoms. In one activity used by Kalichman, Rompa, and Coley (1996), the steps to using condoms from start to finish, from opening the condom package to disposing of the used condom, were placed on printed cards that were used in a sorting exercise. The group organized the sequence of steps, allowing for interaction and discussion about what steps should occur in which order. In another activity designed to address negative attitudes toward condoms, the relative benefits and costs, or pros and cons, of condom use was explored. In this activity, the group first brainstorms to generate a list of cons of condom use that are recorded on newsprint. The brainstorming exercise is then repeated to generate a list of pros of condom use. The resulting lists of condom pros and cons were discussed, reinforcing the perceived benefits of condoms and using problem solving strategies to change negative perceptions.

The same skills building principles used for training male condom use can be applied to female condoms, the only available female controlled barrier method for preventing the spread of HIV infection. Approved for use by the

FDA in 1992, the Reality® Female Condom has been shown effective in preventing STDs and as a contraceptive (Farr, Gabelnick, Sturgen, & Dorflinger, 1994; Soper et al., 1993). Studies show that many women find the female condom acceptable (Shervington, 1993), particularly women who lack power in their relationships with men (Gollub & Stein, 1993). Like other barrier methods, however, the effectiveness of the female condom depends on its consistent and correct use that may benefit from intensive skills training. In parallel to other skills, female condom skills training includes (a) demonstrating the proper techniques for inserting the female condom using pelvic anatomical models; (b) allowing participants to practice correct placement of the female condom using pelvic models; (c) providing feedback on performance; and (d) gaining peer support for efforts to use the female condom. It should also be noted that the female condom has become popular for use during anal intercourse, although the safety and efficacy of this practice has yet to be determined. Nevertheless, HIV risk-reduction interventions have started instructing men who have sex with men how to use the female condom during anal intercourse.

Safer-sex skills training often emphasizes condom use, but its content is usually broader than condom use alone. Exercises for eroticizing safer sex were first innovated by community-based gay men's organizations at the start of the AIDS epidemic. Workshops included discussions and activities to emphasize the pleasures of nongenital touching and the sensations of massage, body rubbing oils and creams, as well as other means of enhancing sensual experiences. Oral–genital contact has also been included as a safer-sex alternative, although avoiding ejaculation in the mouth is often advised. There are many examples for how groups have incorporated eroticizing safer sex exercises into their HIV prevention programs. In GMHC's early program *Hot, Horny, and Healthy*, an exercise was introduced to explore personal likes and dislikes in relation to safer sex. Participants were paired and one member of each dyad was instructed to blindfold the other, taking turns massaging the upper body with lotions and body oils. Similarly, in GMHC's program *Empowering Men*, eroticizing safer sex was defined as discovering erotic nongenital touching and was explored in open group discussions and sensation enhancing activities.

Condom use and engaging in safer sex activities occur in the complex flow of interactions between partners. In the case of women in heterosexual relationships as well as men who are receptive partners during anal intercourse, using male condoms may require techniques for putting condoms on partners and persuading partners to use condoms. Sexual communication skills training therefore constitutes an intervention component in its own right.

Sexual Communication and Relationship Building Skills: Talking to Your Partner.   Sexual negotiation, sexual assertiveness, and refusal of high-risk sex are the most common types of communication skills included in HIV risk-reduction interventions. Many interventions, however, have not clearly distinguished between these different types of communication skills. For example, NIMH's (1995) *Project Light* defined assertiveness as: (1) clearly stating needs; (2) acknowledging partner needs; (3) using I statements;

(4) listening to partners; (5) being respectful and positive; (6) stating one's reasons for personal choice; and (7) standing firm for what one wants. These steps were applied to negotiating safer sex and refusing high-risk sex. Similarly, St. Lawrence et al. (1994) delineated the following elements of communication skills training, again blending assertion, negotiation, and refusal: (1) acknowledging the other person's viewpoint; (2) be specific in refusal of unsafe initiation; (3) provide a reason or rationale for refusal; (4) expresses a need for safety; and (5) propose alternative lower-risk behaviors. Community-based programs also have used similar definitions to guide their communication skills activities. The Los Angeles Gay and Lesbian Community Services Center's program *Life Guard* defined assertiveness as standing up for oneself in such a way that one does not violate the basic rights of others, and stated that assertiveness is a direct, honest, and appropriate expression of one's feelings and opinions. Gay Men's Health Crisis' *Empowering Men* program had participants practice asking for something from a sex partner and sharing with the group how it felt. Participants also practiced setting sexual limits and demonstrating respect for a partner's limits.

At the center of sexual communication skills training is the role play, defined by Kelly et al. (1996) as the process by which group participants have the opportunity to practice skills acquired through the intervention. The scenarios in which roles are acted out are usually derived through experiences with persons from the targeted population. Formative/preliminary research may be used to identify situations in which persons have experienced potential risks. Detailed descriptions of the places, partners, moods, substance use, and other features of circumstances in which persons engage in risky behaviors as well as those in which they have avoided risk form the background on which role plays are cast. Several examples of role-play scenarios are presented in intervention manuals. For example, *Project Light* used the following generic scenes to set up communication role plays:

> You make the decision to start using condoms. Now that you have to bring up the subject with your partner, they say "why start now, we've never used them before?"

> You and your partner get ready to have sex, you're feeling really close and you both realize that you don't have any condoms at home. Your partner says, "Oh just this once, let's not use a condom."

It should be noted that these scenes lack descriptions of settings and circumstances because group facilitators contextualized the situations on a group-by-group basis. Prepared scenarios are also used in community programs for communication skills building. *Slipping and Sliding Dallas*, for example, asked participants to role play the actions of sex partners and friends in various relationship situations, such as in these sample scenes:

> (Scene 1) You have been going out with your partner for 2 years and have lived together for the last year. You have been tested. You care and trust your partner very much and together you have a great sex life. He has not been clear about his sexual past but you are comfortable with what you know. He wants to start

having an open relationship because he thinks it will expand your relationship in many ways. You are unsure of that type of situation and how your partner will act in that type of arrangement. So you will discuss the possibilities with him and also consult your best friend.

(Scene 2) You have been going out with your partner for 1 year. You have been tested and you are HIV negative. You also date several other people, and always have protected sex with them. Your partner has been hinting about having unsafe sex. You are unsure. You talk it over with your best friend.

In place of prefabricated role-play scenarios, some interventions have used scenes derived from the actual experiences of group participants themselves. Kelly et al. (1996), for example, used a group activity asking gay men to write a brief story of a situation in which they engaged in risky sex and another story of when they were tempted or pressured to have risky sex but successfully refused or negotiated safer sex. Although writing these stories served as a consciousness raising exercise, the group facilitators collected the stories that were anonymous—void of any identifying information. The stories were subsequently used in the same group as scenarios in role plays. This approach provided scenes that were more realistic to the lives of the participants. Another innovative approach to role plays was described in the Los Angeles Gay and Lesbian Center's *Project Life Guard*. Group participants were divided into dyads and assumed roles of unsafe and safe partners. The unsafe partner tried to convince the safe partner to engage in high-risk sex. The dyads played their scenario in front of the rest of the group, receiving feedback on the safe partner's ability to stay safe.

Another variation on role plays has used video tapes to create scenes for acting out verbal responses. Hobfoll et al. (1994) for example, used videotape vignettes to present scenes to women in groups who were then instructed to execute verbal responses. In describing a role-play exercise, Hobfoll et al. included the following in their intervention manual:

This (video) segment is a role play demonstrating ways to discuss sexual history with one's partner. In the first scenario, a female will model trying to talk to her partner about his sexual history but will drop the conversation when the partner becomes defensive about her questioning him. In the second scenario, a female will model talking to her partner about his sexual history. The partner will try to change the subject with humor, then with anxiousness and defensiveness. The female, however, sticks to the subject and explains why this topic is important. This will display assertive behavior in a close relationship and using the strength of the relationship as the basis for being able to probe. Following the videotape viewing, participants do a role play and discuss issues of obtaining sexual history from their perspective. (p. 5)

Taking another twist on using videotape for role plays, Kalichman and Cherry (1997) identified scenes in popular motion pictures and edited them for use as brief vignettes in role-play exercises. Popular films therefore formed a realistic backdrop for role-play scenarios. Prelude to sex scenes, that is interactions between couples that occurred just prior to sexual relations, were used to enhance role-play activities for heterosexual men to generate responses. Participants produced verbal responses that were inserted into the stream of interaction by pausing the movie clip and having men say what they thought could be said at that moment to either initiate condom use or redirect the interaction to a safer situation. These alternative means of collecting and constructing role play scenarios were intended to increase the acceptance and interest of participants in practicing assertive responses and were therefore used as the framework for delivering modeling, practice, and performance feedback.

In summary, role playing for communication-skills training must adapt to the interests and styles of targeted populations. Pairing group members into dyads for practicing sexual assertiveness between partners only makes sense in groups where partnerships can be simulated, such as is the case with groups of homosexual/bisexual men or in groups of mixed-gender heterosexuals. Role plays for women have used videotape modeling of sexual assertiveness in scenes that appear like stories akin to television soap operas. Scenes from popular films have captured the attention of heterosexual men to engage them in role plays. What all of these approaches share in common, however, is the opportunity they give group participants to practice communication skills with feedback from peers and group facilitators.

Tailoring and Contextualization

Intervention components are tailored or personalized by including cultural contextual themes that fit the lives of targeted participants. In some cases, entire components or even sessions address issues relevant to the target population, even when these activities are only indirectly related to risk behavior. For example, DiClemente and Wingood (1995) included poetry reading at the start of their intervention sessions for women. Poetry reading was meant to build self-esteem and a sense of self-worth among African American women. Similarly, Peterson et al. (1996) dedicated an entire session of their intervention to address sexual identity and social stigma issues among African American men who have sex with men. Other interventions have woven culturally relevant themes throughout their components. For example, Jemmott, Jemmott, and Fong (1992) couched their intervention for African American adolescents in themes of self-respect, personal responsibility, and developing a positive outlook for the future. Appealing to women as gatekeepers of health in their communities and drawing on altruistic values, Kelly et al. (1996) asked participants the question, "If you had AIDS, how would it affect your family? Taking care of elderly parents, taking care of your children, being able to support your family, having an HIV positive child, or having children removed from your home because you are too ill to care for them." Community-based programs offer many examples of how components of an intervention are tailored to the needs of targeted populations. *Slipping and Sliding Atlanta* (AID Atlanta), for example, placed sexual intimacy in a broader relationship context along with emotional, intellectual, and spiritual intimacy. Focusing on the closeness men can have in their relationships other than sexual intimacy provided a framework for discussing safer sex alternatives.

Despite the universal agreement that interventions must be delivered in a culturally and personally relevant context, there is little guidance for tailoring intervention components to specific populations. Interviewing key community contacts or conducting focus groups with members of the target population is the usual means of learning the themes and values of a community. Tailoring intervention activities may mean using relevant examples, language, and images that will connect with the group. There is also evidence that matching group facilitators to participants along certain characteristics, such as age, ethnic background, and gender may be important aspects of contextualization (Kalichman et al., 1993), but which characteristics are most important to match for a given population are unknown.

Group Process

Group process refers to the manner in which an intervention unfolds as opposed to the activities conducted in the intervention. Process occurs independent of content and contributes significantly to the effectiveness of interventions. HIV risk-reduction interventions use a variety of techniques for building group cohesiveness and bonding among group members. Rotheram-Borus et al. (1991), for example, included deep relaxation exercises to help adolescent group members deal with stress and enhance their coping skills. In addition, candlelight rituals were used for memorializing people lost to AIDS. Similarly, community-based programs such as *Sex With Intimacy for Men* (SWIM-II, San Diego AIDS Foundation) included progressive relaxation exercises for stress management and *STOP AIDS*, San Francisco, included activities for processing grief and loss in their workshops. These activities helped create a sense of shared interest and created a trusting atmosphere in which intervention components could be delivered.

Another dimension of group process concerns the effects of group facilitators and their personal style. Independent of intervention content, facilitators establish rapport, build trust, actively listen, foster self-disclosure, use humor, motivate individuals, and support mutual respect. Group facilitators must deliver the intervention activities in a manner that is consistent with their own personal style. The more scripted and mechanical the intervention, the less pliable it will be in meeting the needs of individual participants. Even in research-based interventions that are delivered with high fidelity and standardized procedures, studies have not disentangled the effects of facilitator skills from intervention effectiveness. Although facilitators in AIDS interventions have often been well-trained professionals who deliver interventions with fidelity, areas outside of HIV prevention have shown that paraprofessionals and peers can effectively deliver successful interventions (Durlack, 1979). There is, unfortunately, insufficient research to draw conclusions on qualities and training that can maximize the effectiveness of HIV-prevention group facilitators.

Drawing from areas outside of health promotion and disease prevention, there have been characterizations of effective group interventionists. For example, referring to group therapists, Yalom (1985) stated that the group leader is solely responsible for creating and convening the group, serving as a technical expert and modeling normative behavior for the group. From the perspective of business management, Schwarz (1994) stated that:

> group facilitation is a process in which a person who is acceptable to all members of the group, substantially neutral, and has no decision-making authority intervenes to help a group improve the way it identifies and solves problems and makes decisions, in order to increase the group's effectiveness. (p. 4)

Thus, the facilitator must be more than an agent to deliver the intervention content and must go beyond contextualizing the intervention. The role of the facilitator is to formulate the group process through which participants experience themselves and their fellow group members.

The importance of the group experience in crafting an effective group intervention can not be understated. Bringing people together who share a common bond to learn about a potential threat to their community can itself be a powerful element of group interventions. The roles of social norms in shaping behavior have been well demonstrated and the small group experience provides a setting in which people can examine their beliefs in reference to a peer group. Allowing people to meet, talk, challenge, and nurture each other may form the most important and yet intangible dimension of group-level interventions.

GROUP-LEVEL INTERVENTION EFFECTIVENESS

A critical mass of research on the efficacy of small-group HIV risk-reduction intervention outcomes has accumulated. These studies have used nonexperimental, quasi-experimental, and experimental designs. Some reports have described innovations or demonstrations of new intervention models whereas others report outcomes from randomized controlled trials. In considering the intervention literature as a whole, several independent scientific review panels have concluded that small-group HIV risk-reduction interventions result in meaningful changes in HIV risk behaviors. For example, the United States Office of Technology Assessment (1995) concluded that; "Interventions developed through in-depth preliminary work with the target population that consist of small group programs that are interactive and include skills development, have been among the most successful at reducing risky sexual and drug-related behaviors" (p. 2).

Similarly, a National Institutes of Health Consensus Development Conference Statement (1997) concluded the following about group interventions, "Interventions are effective for reducing behavioral risk for HIV/AIDS. These interventions should be widely disseminated. Their application in practice settings may require careful training of personnel, close monitoring of fidelity of procedures, and ongoing monitoring of effectiveness."

The strongest evidence for small group interventions has come from randomized controlled trials of theory-based skills-building interventions (Kalichman & Hospers, 1997). Across several populations, these interventions have delivered informational, motivational, behavioral skills, and sexual communication skills training using multiple-hour formats. The protocols for delivering skills-based interventions have varied from as many as 20 group sessions to single session workshops and have produced positive outcomes with several at-risk populations.

Men Who Have Sex With Men

Small-group HIV risk-reduction interventions for gay and bisexual men have demonstrated reliable reductions in unprotected anal intercourse and increased use of condoms. Skills training is typically placed in the context of establishing and maintaining safer sex relationships, eroticizing safer sex practices, and coping with loss due to AIDS. Effective interventions have been delivered to men of diverse cultural backgrounds using similar activities that have been reconfigured for particular cultural groups. Although the outcomes vary across studies, skills-training interventions have consistently resulted in increased condom use during anal intercourse. These changes have been greatest for anal intercourse with nonprimary partners. Studies have shown both increases in condom use and reductions in unprotected anal intercourse (Choi et al., 1996; Peterson et al., 1996).

The first randomized controlled study in HIV prevention used a 12-week session intervention with three booster sessions designed to address HIV risk behavior among gay and bisexual men (Kelly et al., 1989). A total of 104 men were randomized to either receive the HIV risk-reduction intervention or to a waiting list control group. The intervention showed significant and meaningful reductions in unprotected anal intercourse and significant increases in condom use during anal intercourse compared to the control group. The intervention was composed of four central components: HIV risk education and sensitization; behavioral skills training; sexual assertiveness training; and lifestyle changes for relapse prevention. Each component was allotted three of the 12 sessions. Three booster sessions provided support for successful changes and problem-solving lapses to risky sexual practices. Because this intervention formed the basis for many others that followed and because it exemplifies the small group intervention literature, its content is described in detail.

Risk Education and Sensitization (Sessions 1–3). The first three sessions of Kelly and St. Lawrence's (1990) intervention provided a comprehensive overview of AIDS information and risk-reduction information. Modes of HIV transmission, actions that can reduce risk, HIV-antibody testing, sexual risk activities in the context of primary and nonprimary relationships, relative risks associated with specific sexual acts, and dispelling myths and misconceptions of HIV and AIDS were covered in mostly didactic presentations and group discussions.

Behavioral Self-Management (Sessions 4–6). Behavioral self-management skills focused on actions that individuals can take to reduce their personal risks for HIV infection. Skills included identification of antecedents to risk-producing situations (triggers), using problem solving to avoid risky

situations and overcoming barriers to changing risk behaviors. Role playing assisted participants in identifying risks and problem-solving behavioral alternatives. Participants also learned such cognitive techniques as self-talk and self-reinforcement to help guide their sexual decision making.

Sexual Assertiveness Training (Sessions 7–9).   Three sessions focused on assertive and communication skills training. These sessions included instruction in communication-skills and the use of role plays to practice initiating conversations with sex partners about safer sex, produce assertive responses to sexual coercion, and deal with partner resistance to using condoms. Role plays provided participants with practice and feedback on their performance from group facilitators.

Lifestyle/Relationship Goals and Relapse Prevention (Sessions 10–12).   The final three sessions of the intervention consisted of group discussions about relationship goals and personal values related to pride, self-esteem, positive self-evaluation, and health consciousness. These sessions were less structured than the skills training sessions and were more directed at self-awareness and personal goal setting.

Kelly et al. (1989) found that men who participated in their intervention reduced their rates of unprotected anal intercourse and increased their use of condoms. However, in a follow-up assessment, Kelly et al. (1991) reported that behavior change was short-lived for many of the men who had initially made significant changes in their risk behavior. Sixteen months later, 40% of their original participants did not demonstrate enduring behavioral changes. Those who reported unsafe sex were younger, were more likely to be open about their homosexual relationships, and were more likely to use intoxicating substances during sex compared to men who did not engage in unsafe sex. These findings were consistent with change patterns of other behaviors, where relapse to preintervention behaviors is common (Brownell, Marlatt, Lichtenstein, & Wilson, 1986).

Other interventions have delivered similar components as those used by Kelly et al. (1989), but with ethnic minority men. Choi et al. (1996) conducted a single 3-hour intervention session for Asian men who have sex with men. The intervention included four components: (1) developing a positive self-identity and stronger social support with discussions about community values, prejudice, and stereotypical images of Asian men in the mainstream and gay media; (2) safer-sex education—expressions of both positive and negative feelings toward safer sex, providing facts about HIV transmission, and a safer sex game that included issues around different partner types; (3) eroticizing safer sex and condom desensitization; and (4) negotiating safer sex, enacting safer sex scenarios and role playing verbal communication. This intervention was found effective, demonstrating reductions in numbers of sex partners and reduced rates of unprotected anal intercourse. Interestingly, the intervention effects differed for men of various ethnic backgrounds, with Chinese and Filipino men showing the greatest benefits. This finding may speak to the

cultural specificity of the intervention, differential effects of the group facilitators with different subpopulations, or other potentially important factors.

In another study of ethnic minority men, Peterson et al. (1996) found that
their three session intervention for African American men who have sex with
men demonstrated significant effects on behavioral changes in comparison to
a control group. This intervention consisted of three central components: (1)
discussions of being Black and gay or bisexual, the relative advantages and
disadvantages to being a Black gay/bisexual man, building social support,
AIDS and STD information, and large-group discussion of AIDS misperceptions among Black men; (2) enhancing positive feelings about safer sex, viewing
a safe sex video, practice of condom application skills, and developing plans
to use condoms; and (3) dealing with issues of partner resistance, analyzing
one's own hurdles to staying safer, problem-solving safer-sex alternatives,
role-play exercises, maintenance of safer sex, self-reinforcement for behavior
change, and establishing social norms for safer sex. Men who participated in
the three-session intervention demonstrated reductions in unprotected anal
intercourse as well as other positive outcomes.

The impressive changes observed in these interventions for men who have
sex with men provide a consistent picture of promise for the skills-building
model with this population. The promise of this research is somewhat
tempered by concerns about applying aging findings to an ever-changing
epidemic. Studies reported by Kelly et al. (1989), Peterson et al. (1996), and
Valdisseri, Lyter et al. (1989) were conducted in the first decade of AIDS,
raising the possibility that second-generation interventions have lost their
potency with gay and bisexual men, particularly in larger U.S. cities. Indeed,
Kelly et al. (1996) more recently reported preliminary findings from a large,
randomized trial for gay and bisexual men that suggested that behavioral skills
training was less effective at reducing high-risk sexual behavior than a
time-matched intervention that focused on establishing and maintaining
healthier relationships with other men. In addition, community agencies are
finding it increasingly difficult to get men to come to skills building safer-sex
workshops, again suggesting that the small group model has run its course in
many gay communities.

Heterosexual Women

Controlled research trials have tested behavioral skills enhancement interventions tailored for women living in urban areas. These studies have tested
interventions that lasted four and five sessions in duration and all demonstrated positive outcomes with medium-sized effects (Kalichman, Carey, &
Johnson, 1996). Women attending small group interventions have exhibited
increases in HIV-risk-related knowledge and increased personal sensitization
to risk for HIV infection. Increases in condom use and reduced high-risk sexual
practices have also been observed, where in some cases condom use has
doubled from baseline to follow-up (Carey et al., 1997; DiClemente & Wingood,
1995). Skills training for women has emphasized the roles of women and the
differential power they often experience in their relationships, appealing to

women to protect themselves as well as those they love (Hobfoll et al., 1994; Kalichman et al., 1992; Kalichman, Rompa, & Coley, 1996; Kelly et al., 1994).

One example of a four-session intervention for women is provided by Kalichman, Rompa and Coley (1996). In one of the study conditions, women were exposed to the full skills training intervention model, consisting of HIV risk education and sensitization, condom use and safer sex skills training, and sexual communication skills training. The intervention components included in Kalichman et al.'s intervention are briefly described.

Risk Education-Sensitization. This intervention component began with videotapes providing basic information related to HIV transmission and illness. The videotape presentations were followed by facilitator-guided discussions. Intervention leaders reviewed information about HIV transmission and risk behaviors, discussed the prevalence of HIV and AIDS, clarified misconceptions, dispelled myths about AIDS, and described HIV antibody testing. This intervention component included group discussions of how HIV infection is related to personal life situations, relationships, and risk behaviors, as well as individual motivation to reduce risk. This segment also encouraged participants to engage in a personal assessment of their own risk behavior histories and initiate discussions of life-situations that have placed them at risk. The benefits and limitations of condoms were discussed and proper condom use was demonstrated by leaders but not practiced by participants. Methods of effectively cleaning drug injection equipment were also discussed.

Behavioral Self-Management Skills. This component focused on developing behavioral self-management skills related to HIV risk-reduction. Participants discussed personal risk behaviors and cues related to sexual risk-producing situations. Participants were instructed to identify environmental and cognitive-affective cues that serve as triggers for high-risk situations, including mood states, substance use, settings, and sex partner characteristics. Group leaders encouraged participants to think of strategies to manage these triggers through such methods as keeping condoms nearby, avoiding sex after drinking, and remembering information about risk behaviors. Participants were also instructed in the identification of barriers to risk-reduction efforts and discussed methods of removing personal barriers. Condom instruction was also included in this component. Using anatomical models, group facilitators demonstrated proper condom application and removal, followed by participant practice with corrective feedback.

Sexual Communication Skills. This intervention component focused on sexual assertiveness, safer sex negotiation, and sexual risk-refusal skills building. Increasing skills for resisting partner coercion to engage in sexual intercourse without condoms, and increasing comfort discussing safer sex with partners in advance of sexual activity was accomplished through instruction, modeling, and practice. Participants identified past situations of high sexual risk and were instructed to generate and verbalize statements that would have lowered the risk for HIV transmission. Emphasis was placed on learning techniques for communicating feelings and sexual behavior limits prior to entering sexual situations. Practicing communication skills occurred in role play sessions that were aimed to build self-efficacy for talking with sex partners and increasing comfort in discussing sexual alternatives with partners. Sexual assertiveness, negotiation, and risk refusal were modeled by group facilitators and practiced by participants with feedback on performance from both facilitators and other group members.

Other HIV risk-reduction interventions for women consist of strikingly similar components. DiClemente and Wingood (1995) tested a five-session intervention that was developed from social cognitive theory. The intervention sessions consisted of: (1) discussions of positive attributes of African American women, identifying positive African American women role models, and values clarification exercises; (2) HIV risk-reduction information, sexual decision making; and (3) sexual assertiveness and communication skills, role plays with corrective feedback. St. Lawrence et al. (1997) found a similar approach effective with incarcerated women. Hobfoll et al.'s (1994) intervention included four sessions that emphasized information, cognitive rehearsal, role-play exercises, feedback on performance, and imagery for aversive conditioning to negative health outcomes. Similarly, Kelly et al. (1994) and Carey et al. (1997) demonstrated significant behavioral changes following interventions composed of the same basic elements.

The extent to which skills enhancement and small group models of HIV prevention are effective with women outside of the United States, however, has not been tested in controlled studies. Although research in Rwanda has suggested that education delivered to small groups of women following HIV antibody testing may reduce sexual risk behaviors (Allen et al., 1992), the extent to which behavioral skills training would enhance behavior change interventions for women in Europe, Asia, and Africa is unknown. Women's roles in their relationships with men significantly affect the application of behavioral self-management and communication skills training for HIV risk-reduction in various countries. Given their self-directed orientation, it is likely that skills-training approaches will be less effective in cultures that are more collectivist compared to those that are individualistic

Heterosexual Men

Studies of heterosexual men have failed to show efficacy for cognitive and behavioral skills enhancement models to reduce high-risk behaviors. In one study, HIV risk-reduction skills training based on principles of relapse prevention implemented in residential drug treatment facilities failed to show significant effects over and above basic risk education delivered in a therapeutic environment (McCusker, Stoddard, & Hindin, 1996). Kalichman, Rompa, and Coley (1997) also failed to find positive outcomes from a four-session skills-based intervention for inner-city African-American men compared to a four-session HIV-risk education control condition. This intervention was nearly identical to the four-session intervention that Kalichman, Rompa, and

Coley (1996) found effective with heterosexual women. In another intervention study conducted with 1,470 injection drug users, 71% of whom were men, neither a single session nor three-session intervention differed from a no-treatment control group, although all three conditions showed improvement over the 6-month follow-up period (Deren, Davis, Beardsley, Tortu, & Clatts, 1995). Finally, a five-session HIV risk-reduction skills-enhancement intervention for men recruited from a sexually transmitted disease clinic did not differ from a five sessions of HIV preventive group counseling (Branson, Ransom, Peterman, & Zaidi, 1996). Thus, despite the fact that the majority of HIV infections in women result from sexual contact with an infected man, the most disappointing sexual risk-reduction interventions are found among high-risk heterosexual men.

It may be that group-level cognitive behavioral skills training approaches are incompatible for use with heterosexual men. First, men may lack a sense of personal vulnerability for HIV infection because of the differential of risks between men and women for sexually transmitted HIV infection during vaginal intercourse. Low-perceived risk for HIV may be reinforced by educational materials that stress gay men and heterosexual women as identified risk populations. Second, it is unnecessary for men to negotiate safer sex and it is unlikely that many men will refuse to have sex with female partners because they do not have a condom. These behavioral tendencies are deeply rooted in the history of women being held accountable for reproductive decisions and the power differentials that often characterize heterosexual relationships. Finally, the small group setting may not be appropriate for men who are uncomfortable sitting a circle with a group of other men, role playing communication scenarios and sharing thoughts and feelings. Thus, few HIV risk-reduction interventions for heterosexual men at risk for contracting and transmitting HIV tested in randomized controlled studies yielded promising outcomes.

Adolescents

A substantial body of research has supported the use of cognitive behavioral skills training for HIV prevention with adolescents. Interventions designed for runaway street youth, teens in substance abuse treatment, and high-school students have demonstrated positive outcomes, including delayed onset of intercourse among sexually inexperienced youth and increased condom use among those who are sexually active. Jemmott et al. (1992) demonstrated that a single-session workshop focusing on cognitive behavioral skills training produced positive changes among African-American adolescent males, including significant increases in HIV-related knowledge, reductions in risk promoting beliefs, and lower frequencies of high-risk sexual behaviors. The curriculum from this intervention has been packaged as a program entitled *Be Proud—Be Responsible* and has been implemented in a variety of settings including schools and community centers. In another study, St. Lawrence et al. (1995) showed that a five-session cognitive and behavioral skills training intervention designed for teens reduced high-risk sexual activity. This intervention has also been packaged as a curriculum, complete with activities and videotape, marketed as *Be A Responsible Teen (BART)*. *Be Proud—Be Responsible* and *BART* are just two of the many skills-building interventions that have been packaged and marketed for mass dissemination. Card, Niego, Mallari, and Farrell (1996) reviewed 24 such programs that ranged from 1 to 50 hours of contact time. Prevention programs in a box come ready to adapt and implement. However, the degree to which facilitators can effectively implement these interventions and the ability of facilitators to deliver packaged interventions is unknown.

Small group interventions have also been successfully tested in schools. In a comprehensive review of school-based HIV risk-reduction curricula, Kirby, Short, Collins, Rigg, and Kolbe (1995) identified nine characteristics of effective interventions for school-aged youth: (1) included a narrow focus on reducing sexual risk-taking behaviors that may lead to HIV/STD infection or unintended pregnancy; (2) used social cognitive theory, social influence theories, or theory of reasoned action as a foundation for program development; (3) either lasted at least 14 hours or taught students in small groups and used small group exercises to increase the efficiency of time spent; (4) employed a variety of teaching methods designed to involve teens and have them personalize the information; (5) provided basic, accurate information about the risks of unprotected intercourse and methods of avoiding unprotected intercourse; (6) included activities that address social pressures on sexual behavior; (7) reinforced clear and appropriate values and group norms against unprotected sex; (8) provided modeling and practice of communication and negotiation skills; and (9) provided training for individuals implementing the program. Several programs embodying these qualities have been evaluated in school settings in the United States and have shown promising results. For example, Walter and Vaughan (1993) tested a six-session intervention delivered in health education classes in New York City. Based on theories of behavior change and integrating skills-building activities, this intervention demonstrated reductions in risk behaviors among treated adolescents compared to those in control classes. Similarly, a study in the Netherlands tested a skills-building intervention and found positive changes in risk behaviors when analyzed at the school level (Schaalma, Kok, & Paulusses, 1996).

Other Populations

Small group skills enhancement interventions have demonstrated successful outcomes in other studies of populations with high seroprevalence rates. Kalichman et al. (1995) found a four session skills enhancement intervention to reduce high-risk sexual behaviors and decrease unprotected intercourse in a sample of adults with serious mental illnesses. This intervention included four 2-hour sessions of men and women with serious mental illnesses. The groups were conducted separately for men and women, with facilitator teams matched to participant gender. The intervention consisted of the usual four components; information, risk sensitization, behavioral- and communication-skills training. However, because of cognitive limitations that commonly occur in this population, there was an emphasis on essential pieces of information and using repetition in the skill practice sessions. The intervention was found successful, with participants demonstrating significant increased use of condoms and reduced rates of unprotected intercourse compared to a waiting-list control group. Similar findings were reported by Malow, West, Corrigan, Pena, and Cunningham (1994), from a skills-training intervention with persons being treated for substance abuse disorders. Sikkema, Winett, and Lombard (1995) also found a skills-building small group intervention to be effective in reducing unprotected sexual behavior among college students. These studies suggest that skills training for HIV risk-reduction may be generalizable to diverse at-risk populations although it cannot be assumed that the model is universally applicable.

Accounting for the Effectiveness of Small Group Interventions

Small-group skills-building interventions tested in clinical trials have been composed of multiple components. However, few studies have tried to tease apart which components account for the observed effects. Identifying the active ingredients of effective interventions would help guide implementation strategies and inform decisions for expending scarce prevention resources. Although studies invariably report effects of interventions on variables theoretically linked to behavior change, such as risk-related knowledge, attitudes, self-efficacy, behavior change intentions, and social norms, these findings do not tell us whether changes in mediating constructs are associated with behavioral outcomes.

Studies that have addressed the corresponding changes between mediating variables and risk-reduction behavioral changes have used multiple regression analyses to predict behavior changes from changes in hypothesized mediators. In some cases, proposed mediators reflect behavioral history rather than theoretical constructs. For example, using regression analyses to predict behavior change following a skills-building intervention for adolescents, Rotheram–Borus, Reid, and Rosario (1994) reported that sexual risk reductions were greatest for those teens who had lower-risk histories, those who did not engage in commercial sex work, and those who attended a greater number of intervention sessions.

There have, however, been some tests of theoretical constructs as mediators of behavior change. In a study of a single session intervention to promote STD protection among college students, Bryan, Aiken, and West (1996) used regression analyses to show that changes in perceived benefits of condom use, acceptance of sexuality, sexual control, attitudes toward condoms, and self-efficacy for condom use were linked to behavioral intentions to use condoms. These analyses allowed the researchers to conclude that the mechanisms of action for their intervention were affective attitudes toward condoms and condom users, as well as self-efficacy for condom use. In their telephone-based intervention for gay and bisexual men described later this chapter, Roffman et al. (1997) found that positive outcome expectancies, motivations to practice safer sex, and confidence in the ability to cope with risky situations corresponded with reductions in unprotected anal intercourse. These analyses therefore show that theoretical constructs tied to intervention components account for degrees of behavior change resulting from intervention effects.

Although regression analyses provide valuable information about the linkages between constructs and change, they do not identify the independent effects of intervention components on behavioral outcomes. To address this question, Kalichman, Rompa, and Coley (1996) conducted an experiment to test the independent effects of communication skills and behavioral self-management skills building in a factorial design components analysis. African-American women recruited from an inner-city community were randomly assigned to one of four intervention conditions consisting of either: a) sexual communication skills training; b) self-management skills training; c) a combination of sexual communication and self-management skills; or d) HIV education and risk sensitization without skills training. Elements in each of the education, sensitization, behavioral self-management, and communication skills components parallel those described in the earlier sections. Results showed that all four intervention conditions increased AIDS knowledge and intentions to reduce risk behaviors. Communication skills training resulted in higher rates of risk-reduction conversations and risk refusals. However, the combined skills training condition showed the lowest rates of unprotected sexual intercourse at follow-up. This study was the first to experimentally control HIV risk-reduction elements in an analysis of a skills-based HIV prevention intervention. It was suggested that a blend of communication and behavioral self-management skills, as has been reported in the previously reviewed intervention trials, is most efficacious for reducing HIV risk behavior among at-risk women. These results provide further support for the full cognitive behavioral skills training intervention model for HIV risk-reduction.

INNOVATIVE GROUP INTERVENTION

Innovative approaches have been reported that break away from the traditional facility-based implementation of small group interventions. One such innovation has been the multiple session, small group intervention deigned for delivery over the telephone using teleconference technology. Although telephone-based interventions have been reported in other areas of health promotion (Lichtenstein, Glasgow, Lando, Ossip–Klein, & Boles, 1996), Roffman et al. (1997) conducted the first large-scale intervention trial that targeted a national sample of hard-to-reach men who have sex with men to participate in an HIV risk-reduction intervention delivered entirely over the telephone. Drawing from models of social marketing (Taylor & Henderson, 1992), a large-scale media campaign was initially launched in Washington, Oregon, Northern California, and Vancouver, British Columbia, with five U.S. states added at a later point: New York, New Jersey, Florida, Texas, and Illinois. In each location, seven principal methods of marketing the intervention were developed, including posters distributed to businesses and health clinics, newspaper display advertisements, brochures, tear-off business cards attached to posters, press releases to mainstream and gay newspapers, flyers, and fact sheets describing the project. The marketing approaches were multiethnic and stressed the opportunity for men to learn from each other about HIV risk-reduction while remaining completely anonymous. Messages used in the marketing campaign included posters with images portraying hands and arms of persons representing racial diversity reaching for a telephone with the caption "Make the Connection" and illustrations of men of various ethnicities with captions recognizing the feelings of unsafe sex, such as "Afterward, I worry about what I've done," as well as advertisements that conveyed similar images and messages. The marketing strategies for the intervention were therefore developed to target men who lacked access or interest in face-to-face HIV-prevention services (Roffman, Picciano, Wickizer, Bolan, & Ryan, in press). To reduce barriers to attending face-to-face prevention programs, participants were offered the option of remaining anonymous throughout the intervention. A toll-free telephone number was used for the assessments and intervention, providing no phone billing records of study participation.

More than 2,500 men called to inquire about safer sex and AIDS prevention, the majority of whom called in response to advertisements placed in either gay newspapers, the mainstream press, and through professional referrals. Of the 1,834 men who were eligible to participate, 34% enrolled in the intervention.

The intervention was designed to reach gay and bisexual men who lacked access or interest in face-to-face HIV-prevention programs. By delivering an intervention over the telephone using conference-calling technology, employing a toll-free number, and permitting participants to retain anonymity, the study intended to reduce barriers to reaching men who were less open about their sexuality and men who were resistant to seeking face-to-face prevention services. The intervention consisted of 14 weeks of group counseling delivered by telephone. Two trained masters-level clinicians served as group counselors for the intervention that was based on cognitive behavioral skills training principles that included education, risk sensitization, men's relationship issues, behavior modification techniques, sexual communication skills training, and relapse prevention. The topics for the 14 sessions included (1) group introductions and program overview; (2) education about safer sex, condoms, and making safer sex fun; (3) safe sex check-in and goal setting; (4) motivations to change and identifying risk-related triggers; (5) identifying coping strategies; (6) communication and assertiveness skills; (7) more communication and assertiveness skills; (8) Mental health coping strategies; (9) lapses, relapses, and reevaluating goals; (10) social support and peer norms; (11) making and deepening relationships; (12) building self-esteem; (13) lifestyle balance and stress management; and (14) appreciation exercise and sharing future plans. The groups were convened through teleconference calling and men were able to use a pseudonym to retain their anonymity. Each participant received a home resource guide and session workbook with readings and homework exercises. Thus, the group experience simulated that of face-to-face interventions but increased access and removed barriers to attending facility-based programs.

Roffman et al. (1997) reported significant effects of their telephone-based intervention in comparison to a waiting-list control condition. Men who attended the telephone intervention groups reported significant changes in risk behaviors. Twenty-six percent of men who completed the intervention reported engaging in unprotected anal intercourse after their participation relative to 47% at baseline assessment. Follow-up assessments with the intervention condition showed that reductions in high-risk sex and increased use of condoms were maintained over a 12-month period. This study demonstrated that skills-training principles are robust across intervention formats and can be effective in reducing HIV risk outside of traditional face-to-face groups.

A second innovative model for group-level interventions involves infusing HIV-prevention components into existing group structures that have been established for other purposes. For example, HIV risk-reduction information has been incorporated into school classes to reach adolescents (Walter & Vaughan, 1993), self-help groups (Sibthorpe, Fleming, & Gould, 1994), and social service programs for indigent women (Nyamathi, Flaskerud, Bennett, Leake, & Lewis, 1994). Another example of this approach is the infusion of prevention components into support groups for people living with HIV–AIDS. Greenberg, Kalichman, and Treadwell (1996) described the fertile ground that support groups provide for including prevention activities. Similarly, skills-building interventions for HIV risk-reduction have been integrated into substance abuse treatment settings with some signs of success (Schilling, El–Bassel, Hadden, & Gilbert, 1995). HIV prevention interventions that are folded into existing services can capitalize on accessing skilled facilitators, preestablished group cohesiveness, and ongoing group processes. Placing HIV prevention groups in the broader scope of existing programs that focus on other, albeit related, problems opens new opportunities to bringing HIV risk-reduction interventions to at-risk populations. Having captive audiences, existing resources, and skilled group facilitators working in related areas may help overcome the barriers to implementing group-level interventions.

LIMITATIONS OF SMALL GROUP APPROACHES

Despite the consistent positive outcomes observed from small group HIV risk-reduction interventions, there remain several important limitations to these approaches. First, participating in groups does not have universal appeal. Individuals who are uncomfortable in group settings are unlikely to attend these interventions. Second, the logistics of scheduling several persons for a given time, much less to meet for multiple group sessions, poses a significant barrier to group interventions. Research and community experience has shown that few people come to group interventions unless they are given an incentive to participate. Additional research shows that persons at greatest risk may be the least likely to attend group risk-reduction interventions (Hoff et al., 1997; Kalichman, Rompa, & Coley, 1997). Although research-based interventions invariably pay people to participate in studies, alternative incentives such as meeting people, altruism, fun, and food may boost willingness to participate in community programs. Another limitation of the small group interventions is the degree of interpersonal and leadership skills that are required to effectively facilitate groups. Finally, regardless of their effectiveness, the intensity of the group experience requires that only a small number of people participate, resulting in only a relatively small number of persons who may be affected by those programs. Thus, group-level interventions offer their greatest promise when targeted to high-risk individuals in areas with high HIV seroprevalence rates and when they are part of a comprehensive HIV prevention strategy.

CONCLUSIONS

The evolution of small group HIV risk-reduction interventions over the course of the AIDS epidemic can be traced through the following steps: (1) dissemination of basic information in community forums; (2) efforts to sensitize people to their risks, often relying on fear-inducing messages; (3) teaching condom use skills and eroticizing condom use; and (4) building skills for effective communication with sex partners. For some people, information was sufficient to result in behavioral changes. For others, it took inducing their motives to change. Still others have required instruction in proper use of condoms and other safer sex skills. Finally, individuals who have continued to be at risk have required assistance in developing effective communication skills. However, we know that interventions that incorporate all four of these strategies are not effective for everyone and that many people who do respond to these interventions relapse to unsafe sex.

The third generation of HIV preventive interventions must build on the successes of first- and second-generation interventions. HIV risk-reduction interventions must meet the needs of individuals for whom educational and skills enhancement strategies prove insufficient. Heterosexual men, for example, have least often demonstrated reductions in high-risk behaviors in response to skills-based interventions, and may therefore require a different intervention model. Preliminary evidence suggests that skills-training approaches may be ineffective for reducing unsafe sex among persons who have tested HIV seropositive but continue to practice unsafe sex, and individuals who abuse cocaine and other drugs may require specialized treatment as well.

Even under the best conditions, skills-building interventions will unlikely result in long-term behavioral changes for people at risk for HIV infection. Maintenance of change requires ongoing support and alterations in the social environment to promote safer sex. Interventions at the community level have been designed and evaluated that are aimed at altering the social context in which risks occur. Chapter 6 reviews such community-level HIV risk-reduction interventions and their effectiveness.

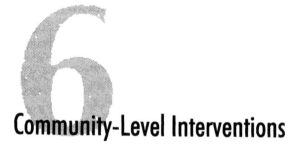

Community-Level Interventions

Community-level HIV risk-reduction interventions go beyond the individual to intervene with geographic areas and entire populations. The potential public health benefits of community-level interventions are therefore apparent; impacting entire communities will have greater public health benefits than the sum of individuals potentially reached through face-to-face interventions. Changes in behavior are typically of a smaller magnitude in community interventions, but the effects are distributed across populations. Thus, in high-HIV-incidence areas, small changes in population risk can translate to significant reductions in HIV transmission. The spectrum of community-level HIV prevention can be summarized in five major approaches: social influence models, school-based interventions, community outreach programs, media-based interventions, and social action interventions.

Community-level interventions vary in terms of their direct contact with individuals. The most concentrated individual interactions occur with social influence interventions, where individuals are targeted and trained to act as change agents in their social networks. Social influence interventions require focused and intensive interaction with a select group of individuals, with the intervention ultimately reaching beyond the original core group. Social action interventions, on the other hand, may not involve any direct individual contact. Social action HIV risk-reduction interventions include policies for access to clean syringes or distribution of condoms in schools (Haffner & Mayer, 1997; Weinstein, 1997). The following sections review community-level HIV risk-reduction intervention strategies.

SOCIAL INFLUENCE INTERVENTIONS

Social influence interventions identify key members of targeted groups and solicit them to participate as behavior change agents in their communities.

130

Social influence interventions seek out persons who are capable of influencing others and enlist them to disseminate an intervention to their friends and eventually to their broader social networks. Social or peer influence strategies operate under the assumption that changes in social environments diffuse to affect individuals far removed from the original intervention activity.

Behavioral changes mediated through social networks spread from a core group of persons to community members, most of whom have never had direct contact with intervention activities. At the center of the intervention is an original cadre of persons whose influence diffuses through social networks, with the greatest impact expected for those closest to the original intervention. The gradient of intervention effects varies as a function of: (a) the degree of influence change agents have on their primary contacts and (b) secondary influences of contacts on additional community members.

The theoretical underpinnings of social influence interventions draw from three major frameworks: social cognitive theory, the theory of reasoned action, and diffusion of innovations theory. In social cognitive theory, the social environment is an essential element in learning processes and behavior change. According to Bandura (1997), behavior has a reciprocally determinant relationship with internal cognitive/affective states and the environment. Continuous feedback between behavior, internal states, and the environment ensures that the social ecology exerts direct effects on behavior. In the case of HIV risk-reduction, for example, safer sex practices are influenced through endorsements of safer sex practices by partners and peers, reinforcement of safer practices, communicating behavioral expectations (social norms) for safer sex, and the availability of condoms. Trusted and credible role models who support behavior change are therefore a critical element in the social environment.

The theory of reasoned action stresses perceptions of social norms as primary influences on behavior (Fishbein, Middlestadt, & Hitchcock, 1994). Subjective norms are formulated through beliefs about social expectancies and personal motivations to follow behavioral prescriptions of specific social groups. Thus, the influence of social norms on behaviors is directly related to the relative importance of persons associated with endorsing the norm. Social norms endorsed by noninfluential referents will likely exert little influence on behavior. However, norms generated by influential others, such as opinion leaders, will theoretically exert greater influence on behavior.

Diffusion of innovations theory has contributed significantly to the development of social influence interventions for HIV risk-reduction (Rogers, 1995a, 1995b). Diffusion theory generally states that innovations such as new products, technologies, and behaviors spread across a population through dynamic change processes. New behaviors are more likely adopted by others when they appear relatively advantageous, compatible with prevailing social norms of a given social network, simple to use, and when they yield observable, tangible outcomes (Winett et al., 1995). People who exert influence on others, often referred to as opinion leaders, as well as individuals who adopt an innovation early play crucial roles in the diffusion of an innovation. In the case of HIV risk-reduction, diffusion theory has been used as a basis for disseminating safer sex messages and messages to change prevailing social norms.

The role of safer sex norms on preventive behavior change was apparent in the earliest community level HIV prevention efforts. For example, *STOP AIDS* targeted at-risk individuals to participate in small group workshops, but the program was embedded in the greater ambition of influencing behavior on a community-level. Volunteers recruited through outreach efforts were trained as workshop leaders and ultimately intervened in their social networks. During the course of the workshop, participants were instructed to tell their friends about what they might do to stop the spread of AIDS. Over the course of time, the intervention dispersed outward until an entire community was virtually saturated with persons directly and indirectly touched by the intervention. Snowball techniques such as those used by *STOP AIDS* are probably responsible for much of the changes in safer-sex-accepting social norms observed in San Francisco during the 1980s.

Kelly's Social Influence Model

Research investigating the effects of social influence interventions on population-wide HIV risk behaviors have suggested promising outcomes. In pioneering research, Kelly et al. (1991, 1992) found that community-level social influence interventions can produce significant changes in behaviors and safer sex supportive social norms. Men patronizing gay bars in three small southeastern U.S. cities constituted the target communities. Based on social cognitive theory and diffusion of innovations theory, the intervention occurred in three discrete steps: (a) identification and recruitment of popular opinion leaders, (b) training of opinion leaders to become risk-reduction behavior change agents, and (c) dissemination of risk-reduction messages by opinion leaders to friends and other members of their social networks. The steps of the intervention, as described by Kelly and Stevenson (1995), are described in detailed.

Identifying and Recruiting Popular Opinion Leaders. So-

cial influence interventions rely on persons who can sway social norms in their community. To identify popular opinion leaders, Kelly et al. (1991, 1992) enlisted bartenders to provide lists of patrons they believed were influential with their friends. Based on their observations and familiarity with the social interactions in the clubs, bartenders were instructed to independently name persons who were most often greeted at the bar, who greeted others the most, appeared well liked, respected, trusted, and who were sought out for advice by gay men (Kelly & Stevenson, 1995). Kelly et al. considered approximately 10% of the bar patrons a critical mass for inclusion as the core group of popular opinion leaders. Once identified, the researchers approached these persons, asking bartenders to introduce them, and explained the opportunity to participate in the project. Opinion leaders were told that they were selected because they were known to be trusted and liked, and that their popularity could be used as a means of preventing disease and saving the lives of their friends. Not surprisingly, few persons refused to participate. Those who agreed attended a series of small group workshops where the focus was on learning ways to become positive change agents.

Training Sessions for Opinion Leaders.

Opinion leaders participated in four weekly 90-minute group meetings led by male and female facilitators. The groups were held in the bar from which opinion leaders were recruited and were framed as social events rather than educational classes. Opinion leaders were not conceptualized or trained as peer educators in the traditional sense. Rather than functioning as information messengers, opinion leaders were instructed in communication techniques for initiating conversations with their friends and strategies for offering their personal endorsement of safer sex norms. Thus, the four sessions were structured as small-group skills-building workshops with an emphasis on communication skills for delivering safer sex messages and establishing safer sex social norms.

The bulk of the first session was spent introducing participants to the intervention, its rationale, and their role in the project. It was stressed to participants that they could serve as change agents with their friends and that it was important that they begin to view themselves as influential in the lives of others. There was also a comprehensive review of basic HIV–AIDS information. It was at this point that participants were introduced to a stoplight image for conceptualizing HIV risk behaviors: red lights representing the highest risk sexual behaviors, namely unprotected intercourse; yellow lights representing moderate risks, such as condom-protected anal intercourse; and green light behaviors representing the lowest risk, including kissing, cuddling, and body rubbing. This image became important at later points in the intervention. The remainder of the first session reviewed ways in which individuals can reduce their risk for HIV–AIDS. This component used the same activities reported in other behavioral self-management skills interventions for small groups (Kelly et al., 1989).

Session two introduced the opinion leaders to activities for enhancing their communication skills to effectively deliver risk-reduction messages to their friends. This element focused on Kelly et al.'s (1991, 1992) model. Following a brief discussion of HIV–AIDS myths and facts, the session turned to the role of communication between friends as a mechanism for changing social norms. Opinion leaders were told that "through conversation you can set the stage for others to be safer" (Kelly & Stevenson, 1995, p. 43). The researchers stressed that opinion leaders should positively endorse safer sex, as opposed to preach to friends. Kelly and Stevenson emphasized using "I" statements and provided several examples of things that one could say to friends to reinforce safer sex as a social norm. Examples included: "Before I consider sex with anyone, I talk to them first—to make sure that they understand the need to be safe"; "I enjoy sex more when I play safe because I don't have to worry"; "When I'm in bed, I'll say no if someone wants to screw without a condom. I explain that I won't do things that aren't safe, and I suggest safer alternatives. It takes willpower, but I feel better about myself afterwards" (Kelly & Stevenson, 1995).

Prefabricated lines such as these were used as examples rather than directives. Session two ended with a discussion of how such statements could be personalized to fit the style of individual opinion leaders.

The third session emphasized sharpening communication skills. The session began with an in-depth discussion of communication, again distinguishing between positive messages and preaching. The steps to effective communication included: (a) stressing the positive benefits of being safe as opposed to fearful messages of being unsafe; (b) emphasizing that safety is the accepted norm in gay communities and that people who are safe are in step with the times; (c) using explicit language to communicate; (d) not preaching but instead using oneself and one's own changes as positive examples of change; and (e) suggesting specific ways to practice safer sex, not just saying that one should be safe. Following several examples of norm-changing statements, participants engaged in communication skills exercises that included modeling, delivery of safer sex messages, role-play practice, and guided feedback on performance. Role-play scenarios for behavioral rehearsal, however, involved discussing safer sex with friends rather than communicating with sex partners. This is an example scenario discussed by Kelly and Stevenson (1995):

> You are out talking to a gay male friend. Your friend sees a guy who he thinks is very attractive. Your friend remarks that he'd like to meet this good-looking visitor and you are sure your friend wants to pick the visitor up. Your friend says to you "I think that guy's really cute and I'm going to do my best to get him." (p.55)

Participants responded to the scenario with statements that they would likely use to discuss the importance of safer sex and communicate safer sex norms. Several examples were modeled and participants had the opportunity to practice in role plays with feedback from peers and facilitators. At the end of session three, participants contracted with the trainers to try to initiate safer sex conversations with at least four friends during the week between sessions. The session ended with each participant receiving a button depicting the same stoplight image used in the educational component of the intervention. Posters with the same image and no labels were placed in the bars. Participants were told that the buttons and posters symbolized the values of safer sex and provided an opportunity to initiate safer sex conversations when they were asked what the stoplight meant. Thus, the intervention placed cues in the natural environment to stimulate safer sex conversations that in turn were meant to reinforce community norms in support of safer sex.

Session four discussed experiences initiating safer sex discussions between sessions and reviewed the steps to achieving effective communication. The session also reviewed information covered in the previous three sessions. Session four ended with opinion leaders contracting to initiate at least 10 more conversations with friends about safer sex and supporting their efforts to reduce their risk. Finally, opinion leaders were asked to think of two people who they believed were also opinion leaders and invite them to the next training intervention. This snowball technique was used to capture overlapping networks of opinion leaders for a second wave of training that repeated all of the components of the first wave.

Message Delivery by Opinion Leaders to the Community.

The mechanisms of change in Kelly et al.'s (1992) social influence model were the conversations between opinion leaders and persons who did not attend the initial training sessions. Although the quality of actual conversations was not monitored, opinion leaders demonstrated significantly greater social skills after the training compared to baseline performance. During 17 days of self-monitoring, opinion leaders reported an average of 6.1 peer conversations in the period immediately following the intervention, demonstrating that the opinion leaders were relatively compliant in delivering health-related messages in their communities (Kelly et al., 1992).

Efficacy of the Opinion Leader Training Intervention

Kelly et al. (1992) used a quasi-experimental design to test the community-level effects of their social influence intervention. Three small cities, Monroe, Louisiana, Biloxi and Hattiesburg, Mississippi, were randomly assigned to receive the social influence intervention at three different time points, with repeated community-level assessments occurring between staggered implementation points. Figure 6.1 illustrates the study design and presents an example of the intervention outcomes. As shown in the figure, each city provided multiple baseline assessments and the intervention occurred across multiple implementation points. A major strength of this study design was that it provided information on secular trends relative to intervention effects. Individual-level change, however, was evaluated because of the lack of statistical power to test for community-level intervention effects.

Kelly et al. (1992) reported significant changes in each city following implementation of the intervention. The percentage of men in each city who reported engaging in unprotected receptive anal intercourse dropped significantly after the intervention relative to baseline levels. Similar patterns of results were observed for insertive anal intercourse and numbers of sex partners. In addition, social norms supporting safer sex increased in each city following intervention implementation. The data therefore supported the efficacy of the intervention.

One noteworthy finding in this study, however, was the pattern of data observed in Monroe. The assessment point just prior to the implementation of the intervention in Monroe showed a drastic reduction in high-risk behavior unparalleled by any other baseline data point and rivaling the magnitude of the intervention effects. In fact, reported risk behaviors remained at this same low level following the intervention in Monroe. The researchers later became aware that one of the most popular men in the community, although not an opinion leader in the study, had died of AIDS during the interval prior to the assessment point in which the decline in risk behavior was observed. The effects of this event on social norms and sexual practices speaks to the impact

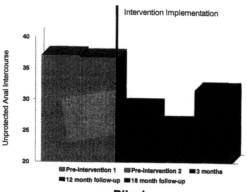

Biloxi

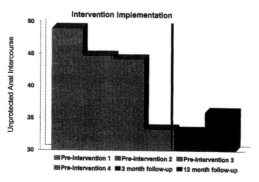

Monroe

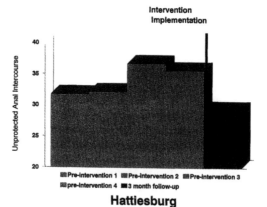

Hattiesburg

FIG. 6.1a, b, and c. Results of Kelly et al.'s (1992) social influence intervention implemented in three Southern cities at staggered intervals with multiple baselines.

of naturally occurring interventions, particularly AIDS-related deaths of liked and respected people.

Kelly et al. (1997) replicated this intervention in gay bars in eight small cities across four regions of the United States. The same intervention methods were used, but the study employed a randomized experimental design with eight matched-pair control cities. This study again showed promising effects of the intervention. The effects observed in the intervention cities were closely related to the number of times that men reported patronizing the bar over the course of the study period. Men who came to the bar more often showed greater reductions in risk behaviors, suggesting that changes were moderated by exposure to opinion leaders delivering the intervention. Important, however, was a lack of differences between some of the experimental and control cities, which may again be attributed to secular trends and naturally occurring events that can overshadow or perhaps synergize with the intervention effects. This possible explanation for the study findings is particularly compelling because of the ever-changing social context of AIDS and the effects of natural events on social norms and behaviors observed in the earlier three-city study (Kelly et al., 1992).

The Mpowerment Project

Another study reporting a community-level intervention designed for men who have sex with men was conducted by Kegeles, Hays, and Coates (1996). This intervention shared several features in common with Kelly et al.'s (1991, 1992, 1997) model, but also differed in several important ways. Kegeles et al. started with a core group of 12 to 15 young gay men who served as the decision-making body for the intervention. The core group named the program the *Mpowerment Project*, designed the logo for the program, and planned social events that served as part of the community-level intervention. In some respects, the core group functioned as opinion leaders in this intervention model. There was also a strong outreach component to the intervention that served two functions: (a) to disseminate safer sex messages in the community in support of safer sex norms; and (b) to recruit men for participation in small group workshops. An ongoing publicity campaign was included in the intervention that placed advertisements in gay newspapers, distributed brochures that reinforced safer sex values, and made intentional efforts to initiate word-of-mouth contacts about the program. The outreach and publicity efforts appeared successful, with over 85% of high-risk men in the community having heard of the *Mpowerment Project* by the end of the study. In addition to community-level activities, the intervention conducted small group sessions. Unlike the social influence model of Kelly et al. (1992), participants in these small groups were exposed to HIV risk-reduction intervention components for individual behavior change with less emphasis on norm-changing communication skills.

Mpowerment small group workshops met for a single 3-hour session that included: (a) an introductory segment consisting of the intervention ground rules and an ice-breaker role-play exercise, (b) group discussion to clarify misconceptions about HIV risk and safer sex, (c) eroticizing safer sex activities, (d) condom use practice on "various dildos and humorous, phallic-shaped objects" (Kegeles et al., 1996, p. 1131), (e) role playing verbal and nonverbal safer sex communication strategies, and (f) informal outreach to train and motivate participants to encourage their friends and partners to practice safer sex. The intervention also included distributing buttons with the *Mpowerment* logo to serve as cues for stimulating safer sex discussions. A total of 168 men participated in the workshops in Eugene, Oregon, the experimental intervention city in the study, an estimated 15% of the young gay men in that county. In addition to small group workshops, community-level social activities were conducted during the study period to influence social norms supportive of safer sex, tap social networks of young gay men, establish interconnected networks, and recruit men into the study.

The intervention was tested by following a longitudinal cohort in the experimental city and a cohort in a control city, Santa Barbara, California. Results of individual-level analyses showed a 26% reduction in unprotected anal intercourse from baseline to postintervention assessments in the intervention city cohort compared to a 3% increase in the control cohort. As one would expect, reductions in unprotected anal intercourse were greater among nonprimary than primary sex partners. Changes observed in the control city were not large and were not in a risk reducing direction. However, many of the changes observed in the experimental intervention city compared to changes in the control city were not significantly different from each other. Thus, although within-subject changes in the intervention city appeared promising, there was a lack of between-group differences for experimental versus control cities. In this study, however, having only one experimental city compared to one control city limited the ability to test community-level change despite the fact that community was the unit of randomization and the level of intervention (Fishbein, 1996).

Social Influence Interventions for Women

Sikkema, Kelly et al. (1996) tested a social influence HIV risk-reduction intervention for women living in urban, low-income housing developments. Similar to Kegeles et al.'s (1996) intervention, Sikkema et al. used outreach, small groups, and community activities to build safer-sex-supportive social norms and reduce individual risk behaviors. Outreach was conducted through the distribution of brochures, flyers, and interactions between project staff and community members. The small group component of the intervention was delivered over four 95-minute sessions. In session one, women were introduced to the program and the concept of being a peer helper. Participants in the groups also viewed a brief videotape of a woman who told her story about living with HIV infection, followed by a discussion about the tape, and then watched an AIDS education video, also followed by discussion. The first session ended with an AIDS risk continuum activity using Kelly et al.'s (1991, 1992) stoplight image and an activity for women to assess their own personal HIV risk.

The second session focused on modeling, practice, and feedback for male and female condom skills and sexual communication-skills, particularly sexual assertiveness. The communication skills training component emphasized women's responses to men's resistance to use condoms. Examples of statements provided in the intervention manual (Sikkema & Kelly, 1995) included:

> This is awkward for me, but I've been thinking it would be a good idea to use condoms. What do you think; I understand, you are right. There is slightly less sensation (with a condom) but we can relax and get into each other without feeling unsafe; and It will be easier (to use a condom) if we practice, and we can practice as much as you like. (Sikkema & Kelly, 1995, p. 17).

Recommended statements even included to convince partners to use a condom, such as, "I trust you, but my doctor says I am allergic to cum, so I always have to use a condom when I have sex"; and "The doctor says I have one of those female infections and we can pass it back and forth to each other, so we should be using a condom to protect each other" (pp. 17–18). These examples illustrate the emphasis that Sikkema and Kelly placed on HIV risk-reduction through improved sexual assertiveness.

Session three reviewed information, behavioral skills, and sexual negotiation skills covered in the first two sessions and introduced the peer influence component of the intervention. Women were informed about the roles of social norms and were motivated to become protectors of their families and community. These themes were carried forward into session four, where women observed effective ways to initiate discussing HIV risk and prevention with people in their lives. Role play, practice, and feedback were again used for instructing women to become peer leaders. Thus, similar to Kegeles et al. (1996) and in contrast to Kelly et al.'s (1992) earlier interventions with gay men, opinion leaders were not sought out to receive the core intervention. Instead, women participated in small group intervention sessions for personal risk-reduction as well as instruction in ways that they could protect other persons they cared about.

Each of the housing developments included in Sikkema et al.'s (1996) community intervention for women organized Women's Health Councils that consisted of a core group of 10 to 25 women who assumed a leadership role in their community. Like the Core Group in Kegeles et al.'s (1996) study, the Women's Health Council was a planning committee for monthly community events that occurred over a 6-month period. Women were given the freedom to develop activities that fit well in their communities and were provided with $500 to fund community events, including educational parties, dances, pot-luck dinners, health fairs, and picnics. The purpose of the activities was to build social networks, provide a place for community members to learn about AIDS, and provide a forum for supporting HIV preventive social norms. The need for creating a venue in which social influence could occur was apparent in the housing developments, which lacked regular social gatherings. Sikkema et al.'s intervention, similar to the *Mpowerment Project* (Kegeles et al., 1996), contrasts with Kelly et al.'s (1992) original model that was conducted in gay bars, a setting that allowed the interventionists access to existing social networks.

In summary, the initial cadre of women identified as opinion leaders in Sikkema et al.'s (1996) intervention participated in a four-session cognitive behavioral skills-building intervention, much like that reported by Kelly et al.'s (1994) women's group intervention. On completing the skills building sessions, the opinion leaders who formed Women's Health Councils assisted the researchers in recruiting successive waves of women to participate in the same intervention. This process continued through snowball recruiting until at least half of all women living in the developments received the skills-building intervention. The small group intervention was couched in housing developments, which also received social norm-changing events sponsored by the Women's Health Councils.

To test the effects of their community women's intervention, Sikkema et al. (1995) randomly assigned 18 match-paired housing developments in five U.S. cities to either receive the community HIV risk-reduction intervention or a no-treatment control condition. Using survey methods, Sikkema et al. assessed women in the developments over a 4-month baseline survey period and then again at follow-up assessment points after implementation of the intervention. The preliminary findings were encouraging, with women in the intervention housing developments showing increases in AIDS-related knowledge and more frequent conversations about AIDS. Women receiving the intervention also reported increased condom use during vaginal intercourse, from 29% of intercourse occasions protected by condoms at baseline to 41% at the 3-month follow-up. For women who reported participating in both the 4-session skills-building intervention and at least one community event, the increase was even greater, from 27% of intercourse occasions with main sex partners at baseline to 45% at follow-up. These changes were in contrast to nearly stable levels of knowledge, conversations, and condom use in the housing developments that did not receive the intervention. In addition, requests for condoms from the project staff were nearly twice as high for women living in the intervention housing developments compared to the controls. Sikkema et al.'s (1996) positive findings suggest that multidimensional community-level interventions that blend small-group skills-training workshops with community-level social norm changing events can result in significant changes in HIV risk behavior.

Community-Based Adaptations of Social Influence Interventions

Social influence interventions based on opinion leader training have been adapted and implemented by community-based organizations. Two programs conducted by GMHC illustrate community applications of social influence models. First, a program was developed and implemented for gay male commercial sex workers (hustlers) in gay bars. The study adopted Kelly et al.'s (1992) intervention model and tested it in a similar multiple-baseline quasi-experimental design. Results of the program evaluation were promising, showing significant reductions in unprotected sexual behaviors between hustlers and their clients, as well as between hustlers and their primary partners

(R. Miller, personal communication, August 1996). Second, GMHC conducted a program for at-risk youth in New York City. The program *House of Latex* (GMHC, 1995) recruited opinion leaders from social networks of gay and bisexual youth who were a part of the house culture, where youth congregate around music, drugs, and sex. The intervention included a four-session training that reviewed basic HIV–AIDS information and skills building for risk-reduction. The intervention included instruction in skills to initiate conversations with friends and partners about safer sex. Once trained, group participants disseminated safer sex messages to others in their social networks in a manner similar to that described by Kelly et al. (1992). This program evaluation again suggested positive outcomes. Interest in social influence HIV-prevention interventions continues to grow, with several adaptations occurring in a variety settings.

SCHOOL-BASED INTERVENTIONS

Schools provide an obvious access point for intervening with adolescents, a population that is otherwise difficult to reach. The need for school-based AIDS prevention programs was apparent in the mid-1980s when risk for HIV infection among adolescents was first recognized (Brown & Fritz, 1988; Brown, Fritz, & Barone, 1989; Howland, Baker, Johnson, & Scaramucci, 1988). In the first decade of AIDS, school-based AIDS education likely included inaccurate information, was sporadically implemented, and was rarely embedded in a broader context of human sexuality. A stratified random of sample of 423 U.S. public schools obtained in the late 1980s showed that 46% offered AIDS education with considerable regional differences; 65% of schools in the northeast relative to 37% of schools in southern states (Wass, Miller, & Thornton, 1990). School-based AIDS interventions face many of the same barriers posed to sex education and are therefore among the most difficult types of HIV risk-reduction programs to implement.

School-based HIV prevention shares many characteristics in common with interventions implemented outside of schools. For example, some school-based HIV prevention interventions only provide HIV–AIDS information using the classroom to deliver AIDS 101 (Morton, Nelson, Walsh, Zimmerman, & Coe, 1996). However, skills-building interventions based on similar principles as those applied in small group interventions for adults have also been delivered in classrooms (Weeks et al., 1995). Classroom-based skills-building interventions may therefore occur in schools but do not necessarily include components dedicated to changing community-level attitudes and behaviors.

School-based HIV prevention programs that encompass multiple intervention levels are usually composed of: (a) curriculum-based classroom instruction that includes skills building, (b) school-wide peer-led programming, and (c) social norms changing health promotion activities. For example, the *Safer Choices Program* utilized a multicomponent, multilevel intervention design to reduce risks for STDs, HIV infection, and teen pregnancy (Coyle et al., 1996).

On the school level, School Health Promotion Councils were formed to serve as an organizational and structural framework for ensuring school-wide implementation of the intervention. At the classroom level, a 10-lesson series for grades 9 and 10 was implemented. This classroom-based intervention was adapted from *Reducing the Risk: Building to Prevent Pregnancy*, a skills-based program with effectiveness demonstrated in empirical studies. The curriculum was implemented by classroom teachers and along with peer facilitators to deliver intervention activities. Students were responsible for implementing activities geared toward altering social norms and school culture, including use of the school newspaper to place AIDS awareness advertisements and run feature stories; school opinion polls to raise aware- ness; public forums and public speakers; small media campaigns that included posters, buttons, T-shirts, drama productions, and rap music contests; and small group discussions on AIDS-related topics of relevance to teens. This multilevel intervention was aimed at changing school-wide atti- tudes and behavior.

Similarly, O'Hara et al. (1996) developed an intervention that utilized peer counselors and educators to deliver prevention activities at multiple levels in schools. The intervention consisted of: (a) large group sessions providing basic AIDS information, guest speakers from the health department and a panel discussion with people living with HIV infection; (b) small group sessions for communication-skills building, role-playing negotiation skills, personalizing risk, and accessing school and community resources; and (c) school-wide activities intended to alter social norms in the school, including an AIDS bulletin board, declaring an AIDS awareness week, information booths, participation in the local AIDS walk, condom awareness, use of peer counsel- ors, and involving teachers in classroom discussions about AIDS. Multicom- ponent, multilevel school-based interventions therefore incorporate individual interventions to promote behavior change as well as school-wide activities to foster community level changes in social norms, activities similar to those used in social influence interventions with gay and bisexual men (Kegeles et al., 1996) and heterosexual women (Sikkema et al., 1996).

In these various frameworks, however, a variety of different intervention curricula may be introduced. For example, AIDS education can be embedded in a comprehensive sex education program that includes sexual–reproductive health, contraception, sexual decision making, and values clarification. Al- ternatively, AIDS education can exist independent of comprehensive sex education, where the basic facts of AIDS are discussed outside of a broader scope of human sexuality. The most controversial aspect of AIDS education, however, is the degree to which the program content covers condom use in addition to information about abstinence. Abstinence-based programs focus on the importance of refraining from sexual intercourse until after marriage. These programs either exclude discussions of contraception, including con- doms, or only discuss contraceptive failure in preventing HIV infection, STDs, and pregnancy (Kirby, 1995; Kirby et al., 1994). Intensive abstinence- based programs have failed to demonstrate reduced rates of intercourse among sexually active youth and have not shown evidence for delaying the onset of intercourse (Christopher & Roosa, 1990; Jorgensen, Potts, & Camp, 1993; St. Pierre, Mark, Kaltreider, & Aikin, 1995; Young, Core–Gebhart, & Marx, 1992). Although evaluations of abstinence-based programs have been methodologically limited (Kirby, 1995), their consistent lack of positive outcomes have brought the use of abstinence-based HIV-prevention programs into serious question.

In contrast to abstinence-based interventions, comprehensive HIV education programs based in classrooms have demonstrated optimistic results, including increased condom use (Main et al., 1994; Walter & Vaughn, 1993) and reduced frequency of intercourse (Walter & Vaughn, 1993). Importantly, no comprehensive school-based HIV-prevention interventions evaluated, including those conducted with young adolescents, showed signs of promoting sexual acting out or hastening the onset of sexual intercourse (Kirby, 1995). These findings are important because concerns about promoting reckless sexual behavior are the most common reasons for endorsing abstinence-based curricula.

Resulting from an extensive review of the school-based intervention literature, Kirby (1995) and Kirby et al. (1994) identified characteristics common to effective school-based interventions. First, effective interventions tend to focus on a few specific behaviors that are most relevant to reducing risks for infection and pregnancy, as opposed to muddying the waters with a plethora of sexual activities that are of low or no risk. Second, successful programs included skills-building activities that enhanced self-efficacy for performing risk-reducing and safer-sex negotiating practices. These intervention components were based on social cognitive theory and included modeling new behaviors, providing opportunities to rehearse and receive feedback on performance. Third, effective interventions included at least 14 hours of contact or were conducted in small groups. Fourth, effective programs used multiple teaching methods and provided opportunities for youth to personalize information. Fifth, although effective programs did more than provide accurate information, basic information about the risks of unprotected intercourse was included in the context of making behaviorally relevant decisions. Sixth, effective interventions specifically addressed social pressures to engage in sexual behaviors and strategies for resisting peer pressure. Seventh, effective interventions were found to reinforce values and social norms supportive of target behaviors, whether the targets were abstinence, condom use, or sexual decision making. And finally, effective interventions provided extensive training for teachers or peers who subsequently implemented the program. These qualities overlap with effective programs conducted outside of schools. However, structural support from the school, teachers, and parents appear particularly important in implementing school-wide HIV-prevention programming.

OUTREACH INTERVENTIONS

The earliest community outreach efforts that described themselves as such were youth employment opportunity centers established in the 1960s (Leviton

& Schuh, 1991). Community health interventions, such as mobile mammography, health fairs, cholesterol screening at shopping malls, and other related programs, are now commonplace and reach out to the public for immediate access to health services. By definition, outreach involves actively seeking people for services by taking prevention activities to neighborhoods, streets, bars, and any other places where people targeted by the intervention congregate (Leviton & Schuh, 1991). Outreach has been and still is a staple in many HIV-prevention service programs. Outreach is not a standard form of intervention, but rather a family of interventions that share a set of techniques and characteristics.

All outreach interventions occur in the natural environment, targeting the intervention to people who otherwise may not be exposed to HIV-prevention messages. Outreach interventions do not impose a formal structure on their target populations. Rather, outreach occurs on the terms of the client. Described as applied ethnography, outreach relies on unobtrusive infiltration of closed communities and participant-observer strategies for establishing trusting relationships with difficult-to-reach populations (Broadhead & Fox, 1990; Kotarba, 1990). The central feature of outreach interventions is their face-to-face contact between outreach workers and their contacts. In this sense, outreach is an individualistic intervention. However, because outreach interventions penetrate communities to achieve community-level change, outreach is conceptualized at the community level. Nevertheless, the face-to-face encounter is the mechanism of action in an outreach intervention.

Outreach provides information and prevention materials, such as condoms and bleach, to at-risk persons in their natural environments. In most cases, populations that are otherwise hard to reach are identified and engaged by community health outreach workers. Outreach workers are trained to enter communities of known risk and become a trusted part of the environment (Watters & Biernacki, 1989), without preaching, proselytizing, or judging the behavior of their clients. Rather, the worker secures trusting relationships in the community and offers themselves as an AIDS information and education resource. In using these strategies, the outreach worker safely and effectively enters social systems to alter the course of the AIDS epidemic by becoming an instrument of behavior change. Therefore, in outreach programs the outreach worker is the intervention.

Outreach interventions, however, differ in their goals and purposes. AIDS outreach activities are most closely identified with efforts to reach injection drug users, sex partners of injection drug users, and commercial sex workers. AIDS prevention outreach activities originated in the mid-1980s as a means of reaching people whose behavior was illegal, secretive, and placing them at high risk for HIV infection (Wiebel, 1993). In these contexts, outreach is considered a harm-reduction service, providing individuals with the means by which to reduce their risks for HIV infection although not necessarily addressing their use of injection drugs. Over the course of the HIV epidemic, outreach has expanded its mission and has been implemented with a variety of populations including crack cocaine abusers, men who have sex with men, at-risk youth, and people living in high AIDS-prevalence areas. Although diverse in their sociodemographic characteristics, risk behaviors, and cultures, many members of these and other subpopulations may be isolated from mainstream public health interventions and are therefore appropriate targets for outreach services.

The Outreach Worker

Community health outreach workers vary in their training and experience, with some programs utilizing professional outreach workers and others relying on virtually untrained volunteers. Outreach workers establish credentials through idiosyncratic experiences (Leviton & Schuh, 1991). The role of the community health outreach worker is a mix of public health field investigator and public health educator (Sterk-Elifson, 1993). Outreach workers must be able to blend into the community in which they are working and be of the community for at least the period of time they are there. Acceptance into the community is necessary to achieve effective outreach. For this reason, members of the target community often serve as indigenous outreach workers who themselves may be recovering drug abusers, commercial sex workers, or of other shared backgrounds with target populations (Wiebel, 1993). Workers are also likely to possess considerable street savvy, knowing where to be, where not to be, and doing what is necessary to remain safe and effective in the field. The foundation of an outreach worker's effectiveness is built on their understanding of community dynamics (Leviton & Schuh, 1991). The AIDS epidemic has created a demand for professional outreach workers whose skills and access to closed communities have made them highly sought after by prevention service providers, health departments, and researchers.

Wiebel (1993) provided a framework for recruiting, training, and employing indigenous outreach workers in HIV prevention. The advantages offered by indigenous outreach staff include ensuring cultural sensitivity of intervention activities, facilitating rapport building with target groups, enhancing the legitimacy of the program from the perspective of community members, translating technical information to street terms, placing the intervention into a common frame of reference, gaining access to social networks, and improving follow-up to reinforce behavioral changes. Wiebel recommended that outreach workers perform their functions in teams and that the team be composed of diverse persons. Field stations may be established in targeted communities to provide a home base for outreach workers. Developing the identity of an outreach worker is key to their success, providing workers with a mission and a distinctive role in the community.

Functions of Outreach

Strategies for identifying and engaging individuals through outreach activities are intended to achieve a variety of outcomes. HIV prevention programs may utilize outreach workers for a variety of purposes, including primary prevention agents targeting persons at risk; in secondary prevention to identify persons already infected and in need of treatment; as a means for marketing the presence of a prevention program in the community; and to maintain low-cost, high-volume HIV prevention services (Valentine & Wright–De Aguero, 1996). In primary prevention, outreach disseminates information and prevention materials, recruits at-risk persons into intensive treatment or other programs, and provides HIV prevention counseling in the natural environment.

Dissemination and Distribution of Prevention Information and Materials. The most common outreach activities are those that distribute HIV prevention information brochures, condoms, or bleach to persons on street corners, mass transit stations, bath houses, brothels, parks, crack houses, shooting galleries, and other places where at-risk persons are accessible. Teams of outreach workers infiltrate communities, offering safe, nonthreatening, nonjudgmental assistance to persons who would prefer to remain invisible. Blanketing inner-city neighborhoods, workers blend into the environment, become recognized over time, eventually trusted, and therefore accessible. The outreach worker is often the only source of AIDS prevention information available to many people at highest risk for HIV infection.

Program Marketing and Recruitment. Outreach workers gain access to some of the most difficult-to-reach populations. They are therefore valuable instruments for recruiting at-risk persons into intensive treatment and other interventions. Outreach workers may inform individuals about HIV risk-reduction programs and opportunities to enter drug treatment. At a minimum, outreach workers may tell individuals about a program or distribute a flyer or brochure with contact information. On the other hand, outreach workers may actually provide transportation to health clinics and social service agencies. Outreach services are only possible through the relationship between workers and targeted clients over the course of multiple outreach contacts.

Behavior Change Counseling. A programmatic approach to street outreach provides sufficient time for relationships to develop between outreach workers and clients, through which effective HIV prevention counseling can occur. Outreach programs distinguish between two levels of intervention: contacts and encounters (Valentine & Wright–De Aguero, 1996). *Contacts* are defined as brief face-to-face interactions or exchanges that center around distributing materials, making referrals, or answering questions. In contrast, *encounters* are defined as intensive interactions in which counseling occurs. All encounters start as contacts, but contacts do not necessarily develop into encounters.

Valentine and Wright–De Aguero (1996) described five elements of an outreach encounter and discussed them in parallel to helping relationships forged in client-centered counseling (Rogers, 1961). The first step in the outreach encounter is screening, where the outreach worker and client make contact and through a brief and usually nonverbal exchange, the worker determines if the potential client is approachable and open to contact. This initial period is equated with the intake assessment in counseling, but occurs almost instantaneously and is based on the worker's street savvy. Following initial contact, there is a period of engagement, where rapport is established with the outreach client. Through expressions of genuine concern and caring, the outreach worker builds trust and paves the way to learn about the client's prevention needs. The third element of the encounter is an assessment of the client's needs, which are elicited from the client and framed from their own perspective. Direct services are delivered following the individual needs assessment and is connected to the needs expressed by the client. Services can include providing information, condoms, bleach, transportation, or contacts with treatment providers. Finally, the outreach encounter includes follow-up, but rarely in the traditional sense of a prearranged appointment. Rather, follow-up in outreach usually involves repeated street contacts where needs are reassessed, strategies revisited, and direct serves delivered. In fact, some HIV prevention programs attempt to develop long-term repeated encounters as part of their outreach efforts, establishing a field-based case management system.

A more simplified structure for describing outreach encounters was provided by Leviton and Schuh (1991), who defined outreach as having three components: (a) establishing an initial contact with target population, (b) maintaining contact until clients become motivated and engage in services being offered, and (c) following up with later contacts to complete the delivery of services. Wiebel (1993) also described similar stages of outreach encounters, including the initial contact, establishment of credibility, and introduction of information and resource referral. Thus, there is general agreement about the structure of the outreach encounter.

Valentine and Wright–De Aguero's (1996) description of the outreach encounter parallels a brief client-centered counseling session and resembles Miller et al.'s (1992) brief treatments for substance abuse. Like Miller et al.'s motivational enhancement interview, the outreach encounter includes an initial contact, assessment, nonjudgmental feedback, and provision of resources for change on the client's terms. Brief periodic check-ins are also a part of both outreach and motivational interviewing. Outreach encounters are therefore individual-level counseling sessions that occur on the street and can mirror effective, brief interventions for substance abuse.

Integrated Outreach Programs. Although outreach programs may emphasize either information distribution, program recruitment, or behavior change counseling, it is also common for outreach services to provide a comprehensive system for performing all three of these functions. One example of a comprehensive approach to street outreach is provided by the *STOP AIDS* model. The *STOP AIDS* approach to outreach used a very brief survey as a vehicle for making contact with community members. People were approached in a variety of settings, including on the street, in parks, bath houses, and bars, and asked to complete a small, single-page survey. The *STOP AIDS* outreach manual (STOP AIDS Project, 1995) described the outreach survey as follows:

The survey is divided into four parts. There is an introductory question to determine whether the person has done a survey recently, followed by a box containing questions to determine the sexual behaviors of the contact. Following this box is a series of open-ended and yes/no questions that are intended to lead contacts into conversation with the outreach worker. At the bottom of the survey is a box containing questions pertaining to demographic data about the contact. (p. 6)

Thus, the survey provides a basis for an interpersonal interaction. Outreach workers were instructed to: (a) initiate discussions by engaging the contact and identifying oneself with *STOP AIDS*; (b) maintain contact by building rapport and securing permission to continue; (c) ask the contact to complete the survey that is conducted as an interview; (d) discuss safer sex behavioral practices when appropriate; (e) determine whether the contact has attended *STOP AIDS* meetings in the past; (f) explain about the program and encourage the contact to participate; (g) if the contact is interested, ask them to complete a referral card; and (h) thank the contact and close the interaction. *STOP AIDS* programs have recruited armies of volunteers who have made thousands of outreach contacts, distributing information, stimulating questions through brief discussions around their survey, referring interested persons to their program, conducting safer sex discussions on the street, and making outside referrals to services.

STOP AIDS outreach workers are trained to engage persons in street contacts and use client-centered counseling techniques. For example, outreach workers are instructed to actively listen to clients, reflect back to a person what they disclose, maintain a professional stance and not develop dual relationships with outreach clients, be positive and encouraging, be respectful and nonjudgmental, use language that matches that of their client, and use appropriate humor (STOP AIDS Project, 1995). Outreach workers are instructed to attempt five contacts per hour, suggesting that the average contact lasts approximately 12 minutes. Much can obviously happen in these brief encounters as is testified by the impact that *STOP AIDS* has had in several gay communities.

Outreach Intervention Effectiveness

Outreach interventions pose numerous challenges to their evaluation, including problems with developing standardized outreach protocols, specifying the elements of the intervention, measuring community-level changes, and complicated issues around obtaining a large enough sample of communities to allow for randomized study designs. Three large scale federally sponsored research trials have, however, examined the effects of community health outreach on HIV risk-reduction. Much of the focus of these efforts, however, has been on reductions in high-risk drug injection practices and, to a lesser degree, sexual behavior change. Nevertheless, these studies provide a wealth of information about the effects of HIV prevention outreach interventions.

The National AIDS Demonstration Research (NADR) Projects.

The *NADR* projects were supported by the National Institute on Drug Abuse (NIDA) to test the effects of outreach delivered to over 36,000 out-of-treatment injection drug users and their sex partners between 1987 and 1991 (Brown & Beschner, 1993; Wiebel, Biernacki, Mulia, & Levin, 1993). A total of 41 program sites were included in the *NADR* projects, of which 28 contributed data for the final evaluation analyses. The intervention sites were located in each region of the United States including Hawaii and Puerto Rico. Injection drug users were identified and assigned to receive either an enhanced intervention or a standard outreach intervention that consisted of HIV-antibody testing and counseling, an education session, and referral to community services. The *NADR* projects showed multiple positive outcomes from the standard and enhanced interventions with certain drug use practices demonstrating reduced risk at 18-months follow-up (McCoy, Rivers, & Khoury, 1993; Simpson et al., 1994). For example, communities demonstrated a median of 21.3 fewer injections per month following the intervention and median of 14.3% fewer multiperson reuses of injection equipment (Needle & Coyle, 1997). However, changes in risky sexual behaviors were far less impressive. Although the projects showed reductions in numbers of sex partners and increased use of condoms were observed, the magnitude of change was small and varied across sites and subpopulations (Trotter, Bowen, Baldwin, & Price, 1996). Data from the San Juan *NADR* site, for example, found no evidence for changes in sexual risk over a 20-month observation period (Colon, Sahai, Robles, & Matos, 1995). Thus, the *NADR* projects showed that high-risk individuals can be reached through outreach efforts and brief interventions can be delivered to large numbers of persons. However, increasing safer injection practices occurred to a much greater degree than did changes in sexual risk behaviors.

AIDS Evaluation of Street Outreach Projects (AESOP).

Supported by the CDC, *AESOP* was conducted in eight sites in six U.S. cities: Atlanta, Chicago, Los Angeles, New York, Philadelphia, and San Francisco. Five sites targeted injection drug users and three targeted high-risk youth. The study design for each site consisted of identifying distinct areas and assigning each area to receive enhancements to existing street outreach interventions (Anderson et al., 1996). The program was evaluated using cross-sectional surveys over time to assess exposure to the intervention, increased readiness to change risk behaviors, and self-reported changes in risk behavior (Anderson et al., 1996). Outreach contacts resulted in injection drug users and street youth receiving referrals for HIV-antibody testing, STD treatment, and drug treatment. Indeed, frequency and intensity of contacts with outreach workers were associated with injection drug users enrolling in drug treatment (Greenberg et al., 1997). Increased readiness to reduce risky behaviors were also found, with injection practices demonstrating greater change than sexual behaviors. Thus, *AESOP* showed promising outcomes from street outreach and was deemed cost-effective in an empirical economic evaluation (Wright–De Aguero, Gorsky, & Seeman, 1996).

AIDS Community Demonstration Projects. The *AIDS Community Demonstration Projects* were initiated in 1989 to evaluate the effects of street outreach to reduce risk for HIV infection (Guenther–Grey, Johnson, Higgins, Fishbein, & Moseley, 1996). Five cities participated, each targeting persons at-risk: high-AIDS prevalence census tracts in Dallas; injection drug users and men who have sex with men in Denver; injection drug users and their female sex partners, and female commercial sex workers in Long Beach; female partners of injection drug users in New York City; and non gay-identified men who have sex with men, female commercial sex workers, and street youth in Seattle. Each city identified two distinct geographical areas for the project. Thus, a total of 10 geographic areas were identified across the five cities, one to serve as the intervention community and the others as comparison community. Each city implemented a common intervention protocol that was tailored to fit the city and target population subcultures. In each case, the intervention was guided by the transtheoretical stages of change model, as well as influence from the health belief model, social cognitive theory, and the theory of reasoned action (Fishbein & Rhodes, 1997). Each site performed extensive formative research to identify the determinants of risk in their subpopulations and used these data to develop informational materials for distribution through outreach activities. The printed, small media campaign consisted of brochures, flyers, and newsletters that were crafted around local culture and served as a major component of the intervention.

The formative research phase was designed to reach persons who would be unlikely to attend facility-based interventions. Each city defined their target population based on characteristics of the local epidemic and prevention needs. It was necessary to determine the geographic boundaries in which at-risk individuals congregated and where the intervention activity could be conducted and evaluated. Over the course of 6 months, project staff performed interviews with local health department personnel and community gatekeepers in each city for each target population. Field observations were also performed in areas where the target population was identified to determine their accessibility and the layout of the environment. The project staff used this information to create localized intervention materials to address the attitudes, norms, beliefs, behaviors, and stages of change of their target population.

Intervention activities were performed by volunteer outreach workers, community interactors, and outreach staff. During the first year of the intervention, over 150 peer volunteers were recruited from the community and trained as outreach workers. Volunteers were retained through team building and social connectedness, with minimal if any material incentives. Peer volunteers reported an average of 27 to 49 outreach contacts per month. Interactors such as health care providers, social workers, store clerks, and bartenders reported 17 to 123 community contacts per month. There were also 22 outreach staffers across the intervention sites who reported an average of 30 to 260 community contacts per month (Pulley, McAlister, Kay, & O'Reilly, 1996). The major function of the outreach contact was to distribute intervention materials and deliver HIV risk-reduction messages.

At the heart of the *Community Demonstration Projects* were locally tailored role model stories disseminated through small printed media including brochures, flyers, pamphlets, trading cards, and newsletters (Corby, Engui-danos, & Kay, 1996; Corby & Wolitski, 1997). Stories were derived directly from members of the targeted community and were presented in materials that depicted firsthand accounts of persons who were at various stages of behavior change. Guided by the transtheoretical stages of change model, each story highlighted motivations, attitudes, beliefs, and behaviors of persons who were contemplating change, ready for action, implementing change, or maintaining behavioral changes. The role-model stories illustrated challenges of behavior change but also positively reinforced contemplating or performing risk-reduction behaviors.

Role model stories were approximately 200 to 250 words in length and included a photo or illustration depicting the role model. The role model stories included information that was of sufficient detail to personalize the model and give him or her credibility. The stories included the situation contexts in which risk behaviors occur, the context of behavioral changes being modeled, the barriers or beliefs that required modification for behavior change, positive consequences for initiating the modeled behavioral changes, and an attitudinal shift toward safer behavior articulated by the model (Corby et al., 1996). In all, over 200 role model stories were distributed in more than 175,000 pieces of literature during the 3 years of the *Community Demonstration Projects* (Corby et al., 1996). Figure 6.2 presents two examples of role model stories distributed in the *Community Demonstration Projects*.

The printed materials were distributed along with condoms and bleach kits in community networks identified by the project staff. These networks consisted of peers, merchants, community leaders, and others who regularly interacted with the target population. Outreach workers recruited identified members of the networks to participate in training sessions that included basic HIV–AIDS education, an explanation of role model stories, and instruction in how the materials could be used to initiate conversations about HIV risk-reduction and positively reinforce efforts to change risk behaviors. The sessions also included role-play practice interactions between members of identified networks and recipients of the materials. The cities varied widely in the number of persons who distributed materials, ranging from 4 to 85 across sites. The number of materials distributed through outreach also varied, from 800 to 6,350 per month. In addition, three cities, Dallas, Denver, and New York, established storefront locations to serve as hubs for the outreach activities.

The *Community Demonstration Projects* were evaluated through self-report surveys administered on the streets of the targeted communities. Using a street-intercept survey method, persons on the street identified as members of the target population were stopped and asked to complete a brief interview assessing, among other things, their exposure to intervention materials and stage of HIV-risk behavior change. Street intercept surveys showed that exposure rates to the intervention materials increased over time, from an average of 9% of interviewed persons reporting exposure during the first

STREET WORKER TAKES IT IN HAND

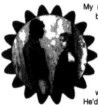

My name is Sharon, and I've been on the streets for six years. I used to have this really violent boyfriend. He's the one who got me started working the streets, and he's the one who got me started shooting heroin. Living with him was pretty tough. He'd act more like a pimp than a boyfriend. He even started beating me up when I didn't bring enough money back from my dates. It took awhile, but I finally got the nerve to leave him. He came after me at first, but he finally got the message that I wasn't coming back.

I'm still fixing heroin and working the streets, but what I have is mine now, and I don't get beat up.

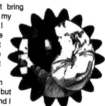

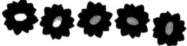

People in photos are paid models   *People in photos are paid models*

Leaving him was the toughest thing I ever did, cuz I was afraid of him. But since I left him, I feel better about myself and I'm more careful about what I do and who I do it with.

Like using condoms. I can sneak a condom on a guy so fast he doesn't know what's happened.

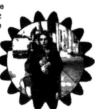

I can do it with my hand or my mouth. I just slip the condom in my cheek, then slip it on with my tongue when I go down on him. Then I move it down with my lips.

I'm not taking any more chances with men. And especially not with AIDS. I take care of providing the condom and putting it on them. So I'm in control, and that's the way I like it.

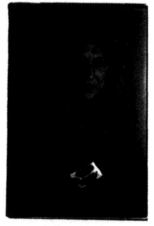

Joanne: Married Women Get STDs Too

I was married and I only slept with my husband. But he was the type of person who all through our seven year marriage was going around sleeping with everybody. Then I got a venereal disease — chlamydia. I know my body, so I know when something's wrong. My husband kept trying to tell me that he hadn't slept around or nothing like that, but I knew he had been sleeping with some girl in another state because he was insecure.

After I got chlamydia from him, I started using condoms. He said he would never do it again, but what if I had gotten AIDS? I divorced him and I'm by myself now, rebuilding my foundation. Now I know that whoever I'm with, I've gotta use condoms no matter what ∞

FIG. 6.2a and b. Example role model stories used in the CDC Community Demonstration Projects.

distribution periods to 38% during early implementation phases. In addition, each intervention community was matched to a comparison community for evaluation purposes. Only in Dallas, however, were intervention and comparison interventions randomly assigned to conditions. In the other cities, assignment of community pairs to conditions was based on pragmatic and logistic considerations. Using a stages of change algorithm to characterize attitude and behavior change (Schnell, Galavotti, Fishbein, & Chan, 1996), results of the evaluation showed movement across the stages of change at the community level, with respondents reporting advances along the stages of change continuum toward ready for action and action following the implementation of the intervention. The effects were greatest among persons who reported exposure to the intervention materials relative to persons who were not exposed. The *Community Demonstration Projects* therefore provide evidence for community-level changes resulting from an intensive outreach intervention.

Outreach as a Social Network Intervention

Social and sexual networks describe interpersonal relationships that link individuals to each other. Networks are important in HIV prevention because they represent the links of the AIDS epidemic chain. Although social networks are most frequently discussed with reference to injection equipment sharing partners (Friedman, Des Jarlais, & Ward, 1994), understanding social networks has become increasingly important for sexual risk-reduction interventions (Morris, Zavisca, & Dean, 1995). Social influence models, the *NADR Projects*, *AESOP*, and the *Community Demonstration Projects* all incorporated networks into their intervention conceptualizations and designs. Opinion leaders, key informants, interactors, and indigenous outreach workers serve as nodes in these networks. Outreach contacts are therefore channeled through networks to ultimately reach multiple persons at risk for HIV infection. Direct contact with an outreach worker, therefore, can have indirect effects on numerous uncontacted peers and partners connected through networks tapped through outreach. New approaches to outreach, partner notification, and targeted message dissemination are incorporating network concepts into their design. Saturating a network of persons at risk for HIV infection with a potent intervention may be among the most promising risk-reduction interventions.

SOCIAL MARKETING

Social marketing interventions employ concepts and principles of commercial marketing for the promotion of ideas and behaviors (Ling, Franklin, Lindsteadt, & Gearon, 1992; Winett et al., 1995). In HIV prevention, social marketing has been used to promote safer sex messages, HIV antibody testing, and condoms. Social marketing campaigns systematically coordinate five key variables: (a) the product, which includes ideas and behaviors; (b) the price, which can be expressed in terms of money, effort, or the psychological demands of adopting the product; (c) promotion of the product through interpersonal contacts as well as media exposure; (d) the place of distribution for the product; and (e) the positioning or niche in which the product fits (Winett et al., 1995). Products that are most often adopted are those that offer greater benefits relative to their costs, are accessible, and are appealing. Social marketing therefore offers tools for enhancing ideas and behaviors along these dimensions to promote their adoption.

Social marketing emphasizes the importance of tailoring product campaigns to fit the characteristics of population segments. Tailoring products requires an understanding of the culture and lives of persons in the target group. Market survey and focus group research are hallmarks of social marketing interventions. Knowing the target population is the basis for marketing decisions and strategies that are designed to meet the needs of targeted audiences (Kotler & Roberto, 1989).

Maibach, Kreps, and Bonaguro (1993) suggested the following 12 principles for implementing strategic HIV-prevention social marketing campaigns: (a) The diversity of the AIDS epidemic will require a wide range of communication strategies targeted to specific population segments; (b) marketing campaigns must be designed to reflect the concerns and culture of target audiences; (c) target audiences must be intimately involved in the planning of the campaign; (d) careful population segmentation is required to focus campaigns on as homogeneous an audience as possible; (e) marketing campaigns should focus on realistic health behavior objectives; (f) multiple communication channels should be used in any given campaign; (g) campaigns must demonstrate that the costs of adopting a behavior are far outweighed by the benefits; (h) social marketing campaigns should be informed by theories of human behavior at the individual, group, and population levels; (i) campaigns must take into account social structures and institutions that influence behavior, such as policies, officials, political, and corporate systems; (j) products and messages must meet identified audience needs; (k) campaigns should have sufficient longevity and should empower individuals to get involved in campaign-related programs; and (l) evaluation of campaigns should be conducted throughout the planning and implementation phases. Coordinated marketing campaigns that incorporate social marketing strategies offer great promise in influencing community-level changes in HIV risk behavior.

Examples of social marketing approaches to promoting condom use are offered by school-based condom availability programs. In 1991, New York City schools, for example, were required to implement programs to increase availability of condoms to students. The program involved assembling coordinating committees for each school that included the principal, parents, teachers, health resource staff, and students. The schools taught a minimum of six HIV-AIDS instructional sessions in each grade and designated at least one AIDS resource center where educational materials and condoms were available. The program also included information sessions for parents. Thus, condoms were promoted through structural changes in the schools assuring that all students would be exposed to condoms and educated about the benefits of condoms. In a systematic evaluation of the program, Guttmacher,

Lieberman, Ward, Freudenberg, Radosh, and Des Jarlais (1997) showed that the condom availability programs resulted in increased rates of condom use among teens, particularly teens that were at greatest risk for HIV, but did not increase sexual activity. Schools were therefore effective in distributing condoms, and the coordinated educational activities likely served as a marketing strategy for condom use.

Condom promotion campaigns also illustrate how social marketing can be used to reduce population-wide HIV infections. For example, in response to escalating rates of HIV infections in Thailand, the Thai authorities initiated the *100% condom program* targeted to commercial sex workers and their clients (Rojanapithayakorn & Hanenberg, 1996). Along with social policies to enforce the use of condoms during commercial sex exchanges, the mass distribution of condoms was accomplished through existing public health systems. Social marketing of the program occurred through a mass media campaign and direct contacts with sex workers. The results of the program showed significant reductions in STDs, including reduced seroprevalence for HIV, demonstrating population-wide reductions in infection rates (Nelson, Celentano, Elumtrakol, Hoover, Beyer et al., 1996).

MEDIA INTERVENTIONS

Media-based intervention strategies capitalize on widespread mass communications to channel information to entire populations (Maibach et al., 1993). The power of media interventions lies in their breadth of exposure and potency of audio and visual imagery. However, widely diffused media messages are limited in their ability to individualize and tailor messages to cultural and social contexts. Nevertheless, information delivered through mass media has played a critical role in national AIDS prevention strategies. Three forms of media have been used in HIV prevention; (a) AIDS informational and motivational videotapes, (b) public service announcements, and (c) publicized social events.

HIV–AIDS Informational–Motivational Videotapes

Messages concerning a variety of public health concerns have been effectively delivered through videotapes. Videotapes that present HIV risk and preventive information have played an important role in educating the public about AIDS. It is known that videotapes are most effective when they are culturally tailored and when information is embedded in a personalized context (Kalichman, Kelly, Hunter, Murphy, & Tyler, 1993; Stevenson & Davis, 1994). When personalized, videotapes effectively educate persons about HIV and AIDS disease processes, HIV antibody testing, behaviors that produce risk for HIV transmission, and self-protective behaviors. However, it is also known that infomercial style videos alone do not produce risk-reduction behavioral changes in at-risk populations (Kalichman, 1996). Several experimental and quasi-experimental studies have consistently shown positive effects of videotapes on AIDS-related knowledge and motivations to change risk behaviors.

HIV-AIDS education videotapes can and do play an important role in broader HIV prevention strategies. Videotapes, for example, serve as information delivery systems in small group interventions, often replacing health educators for presenting basic AIDS-related information. The strengths of delivering information about AIDS via videotape include standardizing information that can be disseminated in a variety of settings, the ability of videotapes to tailor information to a target population, and the capacity of relatively short videotapes to sustain interest and attention. Videotape presentations of people living with AIDS are commonly used to sensitize individuals to their risks and motivate behavior change. Videotapes are therefore valuable instruments for rapidly disseminating informational and motivational messages in standardized formats and culturally tailored contexts. Videotapes can affect negative attitudes toward people living with HIV infection (Penner & Fritzsche, 1993) and can motivate persons to seek HIV-antibody testing. Studies that have randomly assigned individuals to view various information-based videotapes have shown that HIV test promotion messages framed in culturally and personally relevant contexts prompt HIV test seeking behavior (Kalichman, Kelly, Hunter, et al., 1993; Kalichman & Coley, 1995). Unfortunately, videotapes alone have not demonstrated positive outcomes in producing meaningful changes in HIV risk behaviors.

Public Service Announcements

Public service announcements (PSAs) are the most common form of mass media public health information dissemination. AIDS-related public health messages delivered in newspapers, bus advertisements, billboards, and information brochures have become commonplace in most cities. Of course, the greatest media exposure occurs through radio and television. Since the late 1980s, the CDC's *America Responds to AIDS* campaign has produced a variety of television and radio spots. Public service announcements raise AIDS awareness, maintain vigilance against the epidemic, reduce stigma against infected persons, promote HIV testing, and keep AIDS in the public eye. The aim of the PSA is to create a social climate and adjust social norms for either accepting people living with HIV or supporting safer behaviors. National campaigns have produced an array of PSAs, but local community standards and station managerial decisions determine whether a PSA is eventually aired.

In a study of the potential effects of PSAs, the CDC tested two PSAs from Phase V of the *America Responds to AIDS* campaign (Siska, Jason, Murdoch, Yang, & Donovan, 1992). In this study, Springfield, Illinois and Memphis, Tennessee served as test sites for two different PSAs. In Springfield, a television station was selected to air the PSA "Wonderful World," which portrayed children playing in a field and a little girl talking about growing up in a better world. As a comparison, Memphis served as the test site for the PSA "Sofa," which showed a young couple kissing on a sofa while a television announcer in front of them talked about AIDS. In each city, the PSA was aired on one television station during the evening news. A sample from each city participated in a telephone survey, with persons randomly assigned to watch either the news broadcast that included the PSA or a different station that served as a control. Participants were told that the purpose of the study was to assess perceptions of nationally significant issues; AIDS was not specifically mentioned. Follow-up interviews conducted within 3 days of airing the PSAs showed that participants assigned to view the "Wonderful World" PSA in Springfield increased their likelihood of mentioning AIDS as a socially significant issue; more than 72% after exposure in Springfield, as did 54% of viewers in Memphis. A majority (59%) of those assigned to view "Sofa" in Memphis could accurately recall elements of the PSA, whereas 21% of viewers in Springfield could correctly recall elements of the PSA "Wonderful World." This study therefore experimentally demonstrated incidental learning from exposure to brief AIDS PSAs that rival effects of other mass media messages. These findings support the use of PSAs in mass media information campaigns and suggest that PSAs are an effective component of AIDS prevention strategies.

Media Images and Social Events

Mass media coverage of newsworthy events is known to affect public opinion and attitudes (Schofield & Pavelchak, 1985). Media coverage offers considerably greater public exposure to AIDS-related information than most other venues. Media coverage may be planned in advance or it may occur in response to a naturally occurring event. In a study of a planned AIDS information campaign, Crawford et al. (1990) evaluated a coordinated media series designed to inform an entire community about AIDS. The media program was carried out in two steps. First, a 16-page supplement to the Sunday *Chicago Tribune* newspaper featured local AIDS stories and AIDS-related information. One million, two hundred thousand copies of the newspaper were distributed the Sunday before the second phase of the media campaign, a 6-day television news series. Over 6 consecutive days, 5- to 10-minute news segments were broadcasted over WGN television, a major Chicago station. The media program provided factual information about AIDS and improving family effectiveness in teaching children about AIDS. On the first day, the television series was introduced and viewers were provided with the basic facts about AIDS. The important role of families in teaching children about AIDS and in helping children make healthy decisions was also discussed. The second day stressed defining high-risk behaviors for transmitting HIV and ways that families could express their feelings about the facts of AIDS. Days 3 and 4 of the television program focused on the importance of clarifying personal and family values related to health decisions with attention to the health-promoting roles of women and men in various cultural subgroups. These segments included communication exercises to help families develop more effective decision-making skills. Finally, the fifth and sixth days advised families and educators about how and what to tell children, adolescents, and young adults about AIDS and risk behaviors. Again, skills-building exercises were included with suggestions for promoting discussions about AIDS in the family (Crawford & Jason, 1990).

In the program evaluation, eighth grade students and their families from four public schools and three private schools in Chicago were recruited and randomly assigned to either an experimental group, which received a 5-minute introduction to the program and a copy of the *Chicago Tribune* supplement, or a control group that only received the assessments until the study was completed, after which they received a videotape of the program. An examination of differences between experimental and control participants showed that families assigned to view the program reported significantly greater AIDS-related knowledge following the program than did control families. In addition, families instructed to watch the program reported speaking about AIDS more frequently afterward compared to control families, suggesting positive outcomes from the media-based intervention.

Unplanned media events occur in response to a spontaneous news story, producing massive exposure to information about AIDS. One important example of such a media event was the story of Kimberly Bergalis, a young woman who had contracted HIV infection from her dentist, Dr. David Acer, who had also infected other patients in his practice (Biddle, Conte, & Diamond, 1993). The media coverage of Kimberly Bergalis was widespread. Despite the fact that it was an isolated case of HIV infection from provider to patients, the Bergalis case resulted in guidelines for practicing invasive medical and dental procedures published by the American Medical Association, the CDC, and the American Dental Association.

An even greater effect of media coverage was observed in response to basketball star Earvin "Magic" Johnson's November 7, 1991 announcement

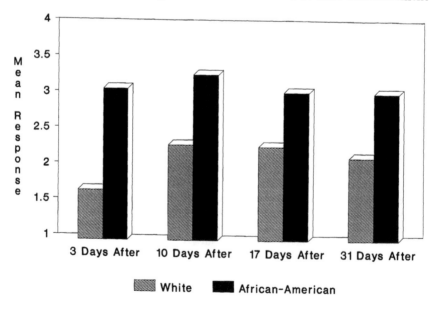

FIG. 6.3. Mean responses for African-American and White men to an item addressing concern about AIDS following Magic Johnson's announcement at four post-announcement assessment points.

of his testing seropositive for HIV antibodies. Kalichman (1994) showed that television coverage of AIDS-related events, such as the death of a daytime television actor from AIDS, the approval of drugs for treating HIV infection, and other such stories result in as much as 40 minutes of total television news coverage across major television stations. In contrast, Magic Johnson's press conference resulted in 235 minutes of media coverage on the day of and the day after its airing, and 150 minutes during the subsequent week. Other studies that assessed quantity of print media coverage for AIDS-related events observed similar effects (Payne & Mercuri, 1993). This unprecedented amount of media coverage may be considered a best-case scenario for media effects on AIDS-related public knowledge, attitudes, beliefs, perceptions, and behaviors. Studies that examined the effects of Magic Johnson's announcement consistently showed significant influences on personal perceptions of vulnerability to AIDS and reduced negative perceptions of people living with HIV infection. It also resulted in increased demand for HIV antibody testing, with some studies reporting a 279% increase in numbers of heterosexuals requesting testing during the 20 days after the announcement (Kalichman, 1994). Calls to the National AIDS Hotline also increased from an average of 200,000 per month to over 900,000 in November and 600,000 in December of 1991. These effects were greater for men than women and greater for African-American men relative to Whites. A community survey among men living in Chicago collected at mass transit stops showed that African-American men were more likely to report concern about AIDS after the announcement (Kalichman & Hunter, 1991), and these effects were sustained over the month following the announcement. Figure 6.3 shows the relative effects of the Magic Johnson self-disclosure on concern about AIDS among African-American and White men in Chicago (Kalichman, Russell, Hunter & Sarwer et al., 1993). Unfortunately, despite the magnitude of exposure and degree of interest in Magic Johnson, no study reported changes in condom use or reductions in risk-related behaviors. Thus, Magic Johnson's announcement produced changes in cognitive and affective domains that parallel those observed in videotape interventions, but similar to the effects of AIDS educational videotapes, there were no apparent changes in risk-related or self-protective behaviors.

The Magic Johnson announcement provides a test of limits of celebrity self-disclosures of HIV infection. Within a week of the announcement, Magic Johnson was the cover story on every major U.S. newspaper, news magazine, sports magazine, and prime time television show. Still, studies that followed public perceptions and attitudes after the announcement showed returns to nearly baseline levels in a month (Kalichman, 1994). Thus, Magic Johnson's announcement left a lasting impression on some people and may have served to remind us that it is behavior that places a person at risk for HIV infection, not who they are. Media events stimulate interest in AIDS and sensitize people to their own potential risks. Such media events may prompt persons to enroll in intensive HIV prevention programs if they are well positioned to recruit newly sensitized persons during the period in which interest is heightened (Krepcho, Smerick, Freeman, & Alfaro, 1993).

SOCIAL ACTION AND COMMUNITY MOBILIZATION

Social action, community mobilization, and other structural changes have been behind some of the most significant advances in combating the AIDS epidemic. The earliest efforts to prevent the spread of AIDS were developed by grassroots gay activists. In 1987, two days following his speech describing the dismal state of medical care for people living with HIV infection and the problems that physicians were facing in getting insurance companies to provide home care for AIDS patients, New York author, playwright, and activist Larry Kramer held a meeting that formed the inception of the first AIDS action group; the AIDS Coalition to Unleash Power (ACT UP). The first and oldest chapter of ACT UP is based in New York City, with spin-off chapters established in most major U.S. cities (Fabj & Sobnosky, 1993).

ACT UP brought attention to numerous social injustices against people living with AIDS, and is credited with several successful policy initiatives, including speeding FDA approval for AIDS treatments and increasing access to health care for persons living with AIDS (Fabj & Sobnosky, 1993). ACT UP has also had a major impact in advocating safer sex practices. ACT UP was among the first organizations to revolt against the concept of risk groups, pointing out that it is what one does, not who one is, that places them at risk for HIV infection. Instrumental in coining catchy safer sex slogans, ACT UP has disseminated HIV prevention information and raised AIDS awareness. The organization is vocal about making safer sex everyone's responsibility, stating that every man and woman should be expected to practice safer sex.

Today there are numerous AIDS social and political action groups. Most AIDS advocates lobby for the rights of people living with AIDS (e.g., the National Association of People Living With AIDS, NAPWA), as well as those directed at strengthening primary prevention efforts (e.g., Sexuality Information and Education Council of the United States, [SIECUS]). Social action as an intervention is responsible for policies that increase access to sterile injection equipment, another example of a structural change with dramatic public health benefit (Weinstein, 1997). Needle exchange and syringe access programs have been proven to avert HIV infections and thus save lives. Policy and politics, however, impede the implementation of these effective interventions. Prohibiting condoms in prisons, reducing funding for drug and alcohol treatment, and mandating low-impact abstinence-based education programs are all counterproductive to fighting AIDS and are therefore frequent targets for social action interventions. Social action, advocacy, and social movements around AIDS have been the most effective means for producing community-level change.

CONCLUSIONS

Community-level HIV prevention interventions target social structures that embed risk behaviors as well as the behavior of individuals. In contrast to individualistic approaches, community-level interventions influence behavior by altering social norms, public policies, and cultural practices. Changes in social structures can therefore have both direct and indirect effects on HIV risk behaviors. Importantly, community-level changes may be essential in supporting long-term maintenance of changed behaviors. Behavior change maintenance is a function of both internal control and external social and environmental forces. The AIDS epidemic itself has been an instrument of change at the community level. The context of sexual relationships has been altered by AIDS. If implemented effectively, community-level interventions can manipulate these existing social structures to maximize the durability of reductions in HIV risks.

7
Technology Transfer

Behavioral interventions have the potential to reduce the spread of HIV. Ultimately, the goal of prevention science is to impact the HIV epidemic by improving the practice of HIV prevention. Thus, scientific findings must reach programs conducted by community-based organizations, AIDS service organizations, health departments, primary care centers, and other service delivery agencies. The ability of prevention research to improve HIV prevention practices has not, however, been overwhelmingly convincing. For example, a study of the CDC's HIV prevention community-planning process, the federally subsidized conduit through which HIV prevention funding flows to the local level, suggests that research has had a minimal impact on prevention programming (Collins & Franks, 1996). The report concluded that after the first 2 years of community planning, there was little evidence that prevention sciences have influenced community planning. One of the study participants stated:

> There is a lot of the feeling around that the emperor wears no clothes in terms of AIDS prevention ... there are a lot of people wandering around claiming they have the answer, but I don't think we do know how to change people's behavior. (p. 4)

HIV prevention technology transfer is the process by which advances in HIV prevention science reach front-line AIDS prevention programming. Technology transfer is known by many other names, including research translation, diffusion of interventions, and dissemination. And although there is nearly universal agreement that prevention research dollars are wasted when findings do not reach community services, there is no consensus on exactly how this should occur. This chapter reviews the state of HIV prevention technology transfer, beginning with a discussion of the dominant models of technology transfer, including their relative strengths and weaknesses when applied to HIV prevention. Next, impediments to moving prevention research to communities are explored. Finally, conclusions will be drawn with reference to a proposed model for guiding future efforts to transfer prevention research to communities. First, however, it is important to define HIV prevention technology as it pertains to technology transfer.

DEFINING HIV PREVENTION TECHNOLOGY

The literal definition of technology is applied science, or a technical method of achieving a practical purpose. In HIV prevention, technology is often used as an umbrella term to cover a broad range of skills, knowledge, and products developed through research and field experience. HIV prevention technology may include developments in condoms, lubricants, microbocides, vaccines, needle access, program manuals, curricula, videos, evaluation instruments, computer software, pamphlets, flip charts, group activities, counseling techniques, and so on. There is, however, a distinction between direct preventive technology, such as condoms, microbocides, and vaccines, and indirect technologies, such as instructional materials and intervention procedures. The former fit into existing structures for biomedical commercial marketing, particularly by pharmaceutical companies. In contrast, there are fewer mechanisms with the financing and infrastructure to effectively support marketing indirect prevention technologies. Nevertheless, the field of HIV prevention is overdue for the dissemination of indirect preventive technologies.

Behavioral interventions for HIV risk reduction in particular have been deemed ready for wide spread dissemination. A National Institutes of Health (NIH) Consensus Development Conference was held in February 1997 to determine the state of behavioral HIV prevention science. A panel of 12 independent, nonfederal experts reviewed samples of the empirical literature, heard presentations from leading HIV prevention scientists, and held open and closed discussions to weigh the evidence regarding the effectiveness of behavioral interventions to reduce HIV risk behaviors. The panel identified several gaps in what is known and pointed to areas that are in urgent need of study, such as interventions for nongay-identified men and HIV-seropositive persons. However, the panel also concluded that ample evidence exists to support the immediate deployment of certain behavioral risk reduction interventions. The panel wrote:

> Based on current research, a number of interventions have been evaluated and are ready to be implemented in communities. Interventions at the individual level include the following: Community outreach, needle exchange activities, and treatment programs for substance abusing populations; cognitive-behavioral small group, face-to-face counseling, and skills building (i.e., proper condom use) programs for men who have sex with men; cognitive-behavioral counseling and skills building (i.e., negotiation, refusal) programs for women that pay special attention to gender specific concerns (e.g., child care, transportation, and relationships with significant others); condom distribution and testing and treatment for STDs for commercial sex workers; cognitive-behavioral psychoeducational skills building groups for youth and adolescents in various settings. At the family or dyad level, interventions include counseling for couples

(including HIV serodiscordant couples) in both the United States and other countries. Within the community interventions include changing community norms through community outreach and opinion leaders for men who have sex with men. (NIH Panel, 1997, p. 19)

An NIH (1997) consensus development panel is a very high scientific authority, and its determination that evidence supports transferring prevention technologies to communities had a major impact on the legitimacy of the HIV prevention field. It became clear that a technology for HIV prevention existed and was ready for dissemination. The conclusions of the panel also provided indirect evidence for many behavioral prevention interventions that have existed in communities for years before the scientific data accumulated in their support.

MODELS OF TECHNOLOGY TRANSFER

Technology transfer is not a unified entity. Indeed, there are many modes through which technology transfer occurs, including program adoption, adaptation, in-agency transfer, and researcher–community collaborations. *Adoption* is defined as the implementation of essential program components by community service providers, with an emphasis on maintaining high fidelity of the prevention intervention. Adoption models hold that interventions demonstrated efficacious in rigorous research trials can be transferred to community-based organizations when there is sufficient support and technical assistance. Program adoption assumes that agencies with sufficient capacity will integrate new programs into their existing structure. This model of technology transfer assumes the availability of adequate resources and agency investment in the value of the intervention.

The literature on program adoption has struggled with the degree to which prevention interventions must be adopted with fidelity rather than adapted to the needs and structures of the agency. *Adaptation* refers to the incorporation of intervention elements into existing agency structures, but with varying degrees of fidelity. Models of adaptation recognize that existing organizational structures and resources often prohibit adopting an entire intervention into the workings of an agency. Adaptation is therefore similar to Roger's (1995b) concept of reinvention, where innovations are retooled to meet agency needs. In addition, adaptation processes allow for the integration of intervention components into existing programs, without the adoption of entire interventions. Although issues of intervention fidelity are acknowledged by adaptation models, a priority is placed on goodness of program fit in organizational structures even when implemented without fidelity.

Prevention technology can also diffuse in an agency, influencing the development of new programs. For example, many AIDS prevention organizations that delivered small group workshops for gay and bisexual men in the late 1980s reconfigured these programs for women in the mid-1990s. Many of the same components used in the men's workshops appeared in the women's programs with appropriate gender and culture tailoring. The spin-off of programs in agencies obviously occurs, but it is virtually undocumented.

Finally, technology transfer can occur through collaborations between researchers and community providers. HIV-prevention technologies that are developed in scientist–provider relationships circumvent many of the barriers that interfere with moving a research-based intervention into communities. A collaborative development by definition means that programs by design have already been instituted in the community at the time of intervention development. Community research collaborations are complicated by the gaps between science and practice, several of which are discussed in upcoming sections.

A number of formal models are available to explain and guide technology transfer. Technology transfer has been defined most broadly as the exchange of information derived from research and development to its users (Rogers, 1995b). A conceptualization of technology transfer therefore describes the channels through which new information flows. Information can move from researchers to users, or from users to researchers, or new information can rise through collaborations between researchers and users. Each of these three possibilities is played out in three dominant models of technology transfer: traditional technology transfer, diffusion theory, and community research models.

Traditional Models of Technology Transfer

Traditional models of technology transfer work from a top-down perspective. These approaches tend to be linear in the sense that information flows down from research institutions to practitioners without formal interaction between the two. In one description of a traditional approach to technology transfer, Blendon, Heimendinger, and Marwick (1994) defined technology transfer as "the systematic process by which research and intervention results are communicated and applied to the health care system and the public; the ultimate goal is to improve health care, and reduce disease incidence, morbidity, and mortality" (p. 556). In traditional models, formal structures are therefore necessary for translating scientific findings to principles for practice. The role of technology transfer is therefore delegated to a third system that goes between the science and practice. At the forefront of HIV prevention technology transfer has been governmental agencies such as the former Office of Technology Assessment and the CDC, as well as government contractors and other businesses such as the Academy for Educational Development.

Blendon et al. (1994) described traditional technology transfer as occurring in six discrete steps: (1) knowledge is derived and linked to an existing knowledge base through research; (2) applied research is conducted to translate knowledge into technology and strategies are designed to move discoveries into practice; (3) new technologies go through a validation process to assure their accuracy; (4) community trials are conducted to determine safety, efficacy, and effectiveness of new developments; (5) practitioners are educated and trained in using the new developments; and (6) widespread dissemination of the application is undertaken in populations. As illustrated in Fig. 7.1, the traditional model is therefore linear and hierarchical.

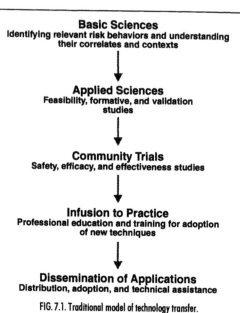

Basic Sciences
Identifying relevant risk behaviors and understanding
their correlates and contexts

Applied Sciences
Feasibility, formative, and validation
studies

Community Trials
Safety, efficacy, and effectiveness studies

Infusion to Practice
Professional education and training for adoption
of new techniques

Dissemination of Applications
Distribution, adoption, and technical assistance

FIG. 7.1. Traditional model of technology transfer.

A strength of a traditional model of technology transfer is its familiarity to the scientific enterprise. In biomedical research, new technologies move through this hierarchy. The linear perspective is also functionally linked to funding structures that operate under the assumption that successful interventions will make their way to communities through the marketplace. Traditional models assume that knowledge is generated out of a need and that when technology becomes available, it moves to where it is most needed (Tenkasi & Mohrman, 1995). The downside of traditional approaches, however, is that technology is assumed to move down a one-way street, from science to practice. Through these glasses, technology is transferred in chronological stages that are not necessarily reflective of the interactive and recursive nature of practice (Williams & Gibson, 1990). Thus, traditional approaches to technology transfer assume that basic and applied research are relatively uninformed by experiences in practice. Traditional models may also create distances between researchers and practitioners, further widening the gap between science and practice.

Diffusion Theory

Similar to traditional models of technology transfer, diffusion theory states that information is generated out of a need and advances are adopted where they will be most useful. Diffusion theory, however, recognizes the bidirectional flow of information that occurs in the technology transfer process. As shown in Fig. 7.2, the development of innovations in diffusion theory starts with a need that is addressed though basic and applied research. Community acceptance, however, is necessary for the marketing and dissemination process to proceed. In addition, diffusion theory discusses the consequences of adopted innovations on existing practices and how these consequences subsequently affect needs that in turn drive future research. Diffusion theory therefore diverges from traditional models of technology transfer by acknowledging the recursive relationships between science and practice.

Gibson and Rogers (1994) described three levels of technology transfer that can be applied to HIV prevention. First, technology can be transferred through knowledge acquisition. Media and information dissemination are forms of knowledge transfer. Second, technology transfer can involve the use of information. Information use supersedes knowledge in that it implies an application. Finally, technology transfer can occur in commercialization, where information is packaged and distributed through interpersonal exchanges in the marketplace. In HIV prevention, the numerous prevention programs that have been packaged and sold, as well as the proliferation of manuals, curricula, and videotapes, represent commercialized technology transfer. It should also be noted that diffusion theory recognizes that knowledge, use, and commercialization can involve innovations that arise through practice as well as research.

Diffusion theory also explains how innovations are distributed through and across populations. Indeed, the spread of HIV prevention interventions over the past decade has occurred in a manner described by diffusion theory. Although other HIV prevention interventions have likely diffused in similar manners, the lineage of small group prevention workshops for gay and bisexual men provides a clear example of diffusions of interventions. The family tree of HIV risk-reduction workshops for gay and bisexual men shown

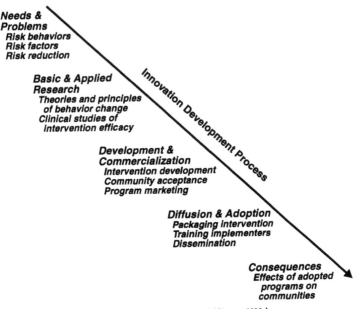

FIG. 7.2. Innovations development model (Rogers, 1995a).

in Fig. 7.3 illustrates how programs have moved across regions of the United States. In a content analysis of program curricula and through interviews with program managers, Kalichman, Belcher, Cherry, and Williams (1997) charted the origins of key group interventions for men. Starting with large educational forums, men came together in AIDS epicenters to learn what was happening in their communities. Soon thereafter, men knew the risks for the new disease but required motivational and skills-building experiences to support them in making behavioral changes. Small group workshops emphasized eroticizing safer sex and developing communication skills for negotiating safety. The first such workshops emerged in New York and San Francisco, and soon spread to other cities with growing numbers of AIDS cases.

It is important to note that the spread of HIV preventive interventions in the community occurred through people rather than an intervention package or curriculum. Descriptions of programs experienced by attendees were handed down to friends and moved through communities. Also importantly, as staff turned over and relocated, program ideas accompanied them to new places. The movement of programs and ideas through relocating staff was documented by Kalichman, Belcher, Cherry, and Williams (1997) as accounting for the lineage of programs. Also shown in the figure, the behavioral sciences appeared to have little if any influence on the development of early programs. In fact, the first behavioral science-based HIV risk-reduction inter-

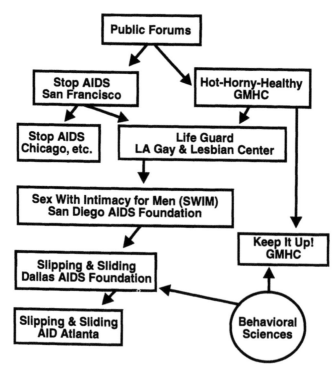

FIG. 7.3. Sample lineage of small group workshops for gay and bisexual men.

ventions did not appear in the literature until 1989, and these studies were initiated in 1986, 4 years after the first community-based small groups interventions. Therefore, innovations in HIV prevention diffused across communities independent of a formal system for transferring technology. Indeed, it is entirely possible that the first research-based interventions were influenced by what had been happening in gay communities. The bidirectionality of technology transfer is embraced by diffusion theory and appears to reflect much of what has occurred in HIV prevention.

Community Collaboration

In contrast to linear traditional models, presented in panel A of Fig. 7.4, and bidirectional diffusion theory (panel B), collaborative models illustrate reciprocity between researchers and communities (panel C). Knowledge gained from researcher–community collaborations may more readily translate to practice because the intervention itself is likely to fit existing community services (Tenkasi & Mohrman, 1995). Researcher–community collaborations have been successfully developed in other areas of social action and disease prevention (Chavis, Stucky, & Wandersman, 1983), but have only recently emerged in AIDS prevention.

Wandersman et al. (1997) described a framework for bridging the gap between prevention science and prevention practice. They cited barriers to collaboration that included differences between science and practice in theoretical orientations, training, funding, resources, and community readiness. However, Wandersman et al. suggested that science and practice can be joined through evaluation, building from the common interests of scientists and providers in program evaluation.

A collaborative model developed for HIV–AIDS mental health services also has application in the prevention sciences. Reed and Collins (1994) proposed a Three Communities Model for mental health research and services that was grounded in community collaboration. As shown in Fig. 7.5, the three communities model brings community-based service providers and people living with HIV infection together with researchers in partnerships for science and practice. Such a model involves shared ownership and collaboration while maintaining independence and autonomy. Reed and Collins noted that joint arrangements between these three partners require compromises from all parties. They also point out that researchers, community members, and service providers each have a stake in collaborating; researchers need access to populations that providers and community members can assure, providers need information from the behavioral sciences as well as evaluation expertise, and community members should demand that research and services meet the needs of their communities.

Researcher–community collaborations offer many advantages but are also met with many challenges. Collaborations require time to cultivate relationships, establish shared goals, and clarify values. Trust is gained only through experience and therefore requires time. The cultures, particularly the language, of researchers and community members can limit potential collabora-

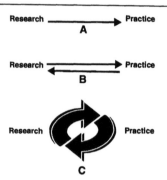

FIG. 7.4. Summary of three models of technology transfer.

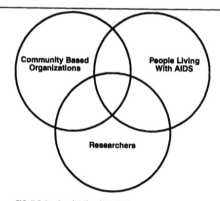

FIG. 7.5. Reed and Collins (1994) Three Communities Model.

tions even more so than disparate goals and values. However, a common language can be established, and when differences in terminology and conceptualizations of prevention dissipate, open communication can foster progress. Issues of transferring HIV prevention interventions with fidelity from researchers to community agencies pose enormous challenges that vary depending on the nature of the intervention and on the characteristics of the organizations involved. Agencies that already delivered HIV prevention interventions may be inclined to adapt intervention elements and reinvent existing programs. On the other hand, community-based organizations that have only offered limited prevention services in the past may completely accept an intervention and comply with implementing the intervention with fidelity.

In summary, collaborations between community-based organizations and university-based researchers circumvent barriers to transferring HIV prevention technology. Issues of community fit and agency accommodation dissolve when service providers collaborate in program development, implementation, and evaluation. Bridging barriers of language, values, and agendas is possible and promotes the goals of researchers and community agencies alike. Unfortunately, despite their apparent advantages and the potential for collaborative models to expedite technology transfer, there have been few such collaborative models in HIV prevention. The paucity of research–community collaborations may be attributed to the difficulties in forming such relationships.

IMPEDIMENTS TO HIV PREVENTION TECHNOLOGY TRANSFER

Transferring knowledge gained from research to communities is impeded by differences between scientists and practitioners in terms of values, language, and purposes. The gap between science and practice amounts to nothing less than a cultural divide. Beutler, Williams, Wakefield, and Entwistle (1995) indicated that science-practice differences are nearly universal, citing examples from mental health, nursing, medicine, and dentistry. Beutler et al. summarized the science-practice split in the following passage:

> In virtually every discipline in which the usual access to knowledge is through the scientific method, scientists have lamented that practitioners are inadequately trained, are insensitive to the values of scientific findings, and fail to read the right journals. Conversely, practitioners are dismayed because scientists offer too little, are consumed by irrelevant questions, and fail to appreciate the knowledge that arises from practice. (p. 985)

Supporting the universality described by Beutler et al. (1995) are experiences in HIV prevention. HIV prevention scientists and practitioners have spoken different languages throughout the epidemic. Researchers use such terms as determinants of behavior, principles of behavior change, and mediators of intervention outcomes. Community service providers want to know what works and how to implement programs that do work. Researchers speak of interventions and providers refer to programs. Researchers pay their participants for their time, affording them access to people who would never come to community service programs. The goal of research is to produce papers published in peer-refereed journals, whereas the product of programs is in the assurance of continued resources to sustain services (Altman, 1995). These very basic differences are at the root of many barriers between HIV prevention researchers and prevention programs.

Brown (1995) described five significant barriers to transferring drug abuse treatment programs from research to communities that also apply to HIV prevention technology transfer: relevance, timeliness, clarity, credibility, and acceptability. There are additional issues of intervention ownership, fidelity, generalizability, and agency capacity that create barriers to HIV prevention technology transfer, each of which is briefly discussed next.

Relevance

Intervention technologies that do not fit communities and lack personal relevance to targeted individuals will be rejected by community providers and members. Interventions run the greatest risk of being irrelevant when they are handed down to front-line practitioners by an authoritarian system. Including practitioners in the planning and development of an intervention will foster relevance (Brown, 1995). Traditional models of technology transfer offer the least opportunity for such collaborations and are therefore at the greatest risk for delivering irrelevant interventions.

Timeliness

Interventions are developed out of a need, and in the case of HIV prevention, the need is urgent. In addition, the needs HIV prevention interventions address are constantly changing. Thus, the relatively slow pace of science creates another barrier to transferring knowledge to communities. The methodical demands of research are far outpaced by the HIV epidemic. For example, the first studies to prevent HIV infection among gay men were conducted in 1987, were published in 1989, and disseminated in 1990. Unlike community programs, research protocols are not revised during their implementation to meet the changing needs of communities. Community programs undergo continuous revision throughout their existence. Just as the epidemic has changed over the years, so too have the programs offered by communities. But research requires years, operating on 4 or 5 year grant cycles, with years added by publication lags, further slowing the dissemination of research findings.

Clarity

Brown (1995) discussed *clarity* as "using a language and format that make findings accessible" (p. 172). Reliance on professional journals for the dissemination of research results impedes the transfer of knowledge. Countless studies have shown that practitioners value scientific progress, but they do not access advances in their field through the scientific literature. Beutler et al. (1995), for example, surveyed mental health professionals and found that clinicians valued research but were more likely to read books, newsletters, and clinicians' digests to learn of scientific advances. Similar findings have been reported in AIDS prevention services. Goldstein, Wrubel, Faigeles, and DeCarlo (1996) interviewed program managers of AIDS prevention programs and found that although 97% had accessed information from scientific publications, only 42% viewed scientific outlets as very important sources of information. The most valued sources were colleagues and collaborators, illustrating the importance of interpersonal relationships in transferring technology to providers.

There are probably many reasons why the research literature is not an adequate means for communicating advances in prevention sciences to prevention practitioners. Collins and Franks (1996) identified eight key barriers to using information disseminated through published research; academic language, length, theoretical nature, unclear transferability, outdated information, lack of information on unsuccessful interventions, failure to describe details of intervention content, and gaps in research on specific problems. Scientific publications may therefore facilitate communication among scientists and create a repository for scientific advances, but research articles cannot be considered a means of directly advancing the state of prevention practice.

Credibility

Research findings and researchers must be viewed as credible if scientific findings are to have any impact on community practices (Brown, 1995). The credibility of HIV prevention researchers is compromised when investigators claim to succeed in preventing HIV simply because their interventions are based on theory, rigor, or careful evaluation. Informal theories used by community providers are backed up by their experiences. Providers will therefore resent the arrogance of far removed researchers staking claims of knowing better what to do to reduce risks in their community.

Acceptability

Providers are often unwilling to accept innovations because of the state of their practice. Organizational change can be resisted simply because change is hard. New programs may not be adopted in an effort to maintain the status quo (Brown, 1995). Thus, pieces of particular technologies will more likely be infused into existing programs rather than assimilating entirely new interventions into an agency structure. Traditional models of technology transfer operate under the assumption that agencies will adopt new interventions wholesale, an assumption that is not born out in practice.

Ownership

Program adoption is more likely when agencies have a vested interest in its success. Tied to ownership are issues of power and control (Altman, 1995). Developing a program from its inception increases the odds that it will fit the identity of the adopting agency. In addition, programs with increased community ownership are more likely to be implemented and sustained (Wandersman et al., 1997). Thus, community ownership is cultivated through direct involvement in intervention development.

Fidelity

That community-based agencies should adopt HIV prevention interventions with fidelity is often advised by researchers. Interventions validated through research are expected to produce results only when adopted in close proximity to the original model (Blakely et al., 1987). Thus, a prescriptive approach to interventions requires careful attention to fidelity. In fact, the importance of fidelity in program adoption was stated clearly by the NIH (1997) Consensus Development Conference panel:

> A critical issue that must be addressed involves the criteria for choosing interventions most ready for implementation in the community. The most obvious is evidence of strong effects observed under rigorous, controlled research

conditions. Among programs with strong effects, priority should be given to interventions that can be delivered with high reliability and fidelity to the original program model. (p. 22)

It is important to note, however, that the panel's emphasis on adoption with fidelity represented a traditional view of technology transfer, as one would expect from an NIH panel, that was not grounded in empirical evidence and probably does not fit well in the HIV behavioral prevention arena. Indeed, there are alternative approaches that de-emphasize the importance of fidelity. For example, diffusion theory (Rogers, 1995a) stressed the reinvention of interventions in existing practices. Although mechanisms of action can be retained in reinvention, there is little guidance for how to preserve principles of behavior change when reinventing HIV risk-reduction interventions. Although questions of fidelity can be addressed through empirical study, there has been surprisingly little research in establishing issues of fidelity in AIDS prevention interventions.

Generalizability

The results of HIV prevention research are obtained under optimal conditions that have little resemblance to the real world of service settings. Researchers are generally well financed for marketing, recruiting participants, and implementing interventions. Most notably, researchers are capable of inducing persons to participate with cash incentive payments, a resource community service providers rarely have.

Researchers are aware of the limitations that incentive payments place on the generalizability of their findings. In a study of injection drug users and their sex partners, Deren, Stephens, Davis, Feucht, and Tortu (1994) showed that monetary incentives, as opposed to food coupons or gift certificates, result in increased attendance to HIV-prevention group sessions. The type of incentive offered was also significantly related to completion of the intervention. These findings support anecdotal accounts from both researchers and community agencies indicating that few people will come to HIV prevention interventions without an external source of motivation. Thus, research supports using monetary incentives to induce participation in multiple session HIV prevention interventions as a potentially cost-effective means of attracting individuals to services. Funders should therefore be persuaded to support providing incentive payments to attract initial intervention participation. For example, the U.S. Conference of Mayors has supported cash incentives to induce men who have sex with men to participate in community-based HIV prevention workshops (R. Carne, personal communication, 1996).

Capacity

The disparity between resources required to implement research-based prevention interventions in community settings and resources available to service providers can bring HIV-prevention technology transfer to a screeching halt. Capacity building must therefore precede efforts to transfer prevention technology to communities. Although there are many dimensions of agency capacity for adopting prevention interventions, few seem as vital as retaining skilled interventionists to conduct program activities. In the first place, community-based agencies often lack sufficient staff to meet their daily programmatic needs. In addition, staff turnover is notoriously high among AIDS service organizations. It is also likely that community-based interventionists will not be experienced or trained for delivering behavioral interventions, particularly those conducted in small group workshops. There are currently no guidelines for selecting or training effective HIV-risk reduction group facilitators. Skills used in facilitating business meetings, working groups, focus groups, or even group therapy are inherently different from those required for blending public health and mental health models for HIV prevention interventions. Cultivating talents and training in techniques for effective HIV-risk reduction intervention facilitation must be a priority in efforts to transfer HIV prevention technologies to community settings.

COSTS AND BENEFITS OF PREVENTION

Cost effectiveness analyses are valuable in setting HIV prevention policies and establishing decision criteria for intervention dissemination. HIV prevention resources are relatively scarce and funding decisions require careful consideration of which interventions offer the greatest promise relative to their costs. Cost-effectiveness studies model such items as salaries, intervention materials, and client transportation against the value of averted HIV infections, usually stated in terms of medical costs and quality-adjusted life years saved.

Economic analyses have shown that HIV prevention interventions are cost effective, and many are actually cost-saving (Holtgrave et al., 1995). Such interventions as screening for HIV infection in acute care settings (Owens, Nease, & Harris, 1996), HIV testing and counseling programs (Holtgrave, Valdiserri, Gerber, & Hinman, 1993) and small group interventions including Valdiserri, Lyter et al.'s (1989) risk reduction workshop (Pinkerton, Holtgrave, & Valdiserri, 1997) and Kelly et al.'s (1989) cognitive–behavioral risk-reduction intervention for men who have sex with men (Holtgrave & Kelly, 1997) have all demonstrated cost effectiveness under a range of estimates and assumptions. For example, Holtgrave and Kelly (1996) examined the cost effectiveness of Kelly et al.'s (1994) cognitive–behavioral group intervention for inner-city women and found that the intervention cost $269 per client served with an estimated .38 HIV infections averted. This translates to a cost-utility ratio of approximately $2,000 per discounted quality adjusted years of life saved, deemed to be favorable compared to other life-saving interventions. Holtgrave and Kelly (1996) cautioned that the results of their analyses were limited by some of their assumptions. However, taken together, the results of cost-effectiveness studies suggest that HIV prevention is money well spent and supports societal efforts to transfer these technologies to communities.

IMPROVING HIV PREVENTION
TECHNOLOGY TRANSFER

Many of the barriers to HIV prevention technology transfer can be addressed by changing how research and communities relate to each other. Figure 7.6 presents a model first described by Kalichman, Belcher, Cherry, and Williams (1997) that links research to communities in such a way that theoretical hypotheses can generate meaningful studies that, with rapid turn-around, make interventions available for immediate transfer to communities. Theories of HIV risk reduction must be responsive to changes in the HIV epidemic and community needs and research must reflect issues in the current state of the epidemic. Studies must also rapidly turn around results to communities. HIV prevention studies are typically funded through mechanisms that result in as much as 5 years of support for a single study that can then take an additional 2 years to appear in the literature. Community providers accurately view scientific advances as late in the game and out of synch with current needs. These gaps between scientific outcomes and community programs can cause resentment toward researchers due to the impression of wasting precious prevention resources.

There are changes that could facilitate the transfer of prevention technology to communities. Research funding structures and research designs, for example, that focus on effect sizes rather than statistical probabilities can help reduce the pressure for large samples, and therefore reduce the time needed to conduct an intervention study. Once completed, the results of prevention trials must be transferable to communities. Achieving a common language and value system that researchers and community programmers share requires time. There are, however, inroads to facilitating collaborations. First, community-based behavioral scientists, such as program evaluators and researchers working in community agencies, can serve as translators to bridge the cultural differences between researchers and providers (Kalichman, Belcher, Cherry,

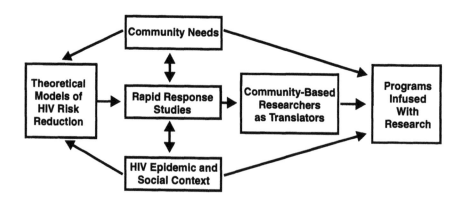

FIG. 7.6. Kalichman et al.'s (1997) proposed model for HIV prevention technology transfer.

& Williams, 1997; Wandersman et al. 1997). Similarly, consultation from community providers to researchers will lead to more relevant research questions and ecologically valid studies.

The CDC community planning process also offers a structure for infusing HIV prevention research into prevention services. Since 1994, the CDC has worked with state health departments to restructure federally sponsored HIV prevention activities. Among the principles of HIV prevention community planning, it is specified that priorities are to be set for intervention strategies based on documented need, science, consumer preferences, and local circumstances (Valdiserri, Aultman, & Curran, 1995). The official guidance for community planning also states that interventions based on theories of behavior change or social change should be given priority in planning prevention activities. The CDC offers technical assistance to state community planning councils for infusing behavioral sciences into prevention planning. Community planning therefore provides a framework in which behavioral science and community practitioner partnerships can be forged and can ultimately facilitate the transfer of HIV prevention technologies to communities.

CONCLUSIONS

Unlike other health behavior problems where science has led the way through research and development to provide prevention technologies for application, AIDS first mobilized communities to address needs before prevention researchers arrived on the scene. Although working to achieve similar goals, researchers and community program developers often do not share common values, language, or paradigms. Advances such as the NIH Consensus Development Conference on HIV Behavioral Interventions, which defined technologies available for dissemination, and the CDC's community planning initiative, which provides a structure for funneling interventions to communities, create optimism for the future of HIV prevention technology transfer.

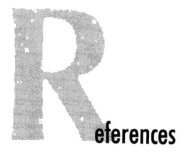
References

Ajzen, I. (1988). *Attitudes, personality, and behavior.* Chicago: Dorsey.

Ajzen, I., & Fishbein, M. (1980). *Understanding attitudes and predicting social behavior.* Englewood Cliffs, NJ: Prentice–Hall.

Ajzen, I. & Madden, T. (1986). Prediction of goal-directed behaviour: Attitudes, intentions, and perceived behavioral control. *Journal of Experimental Social Psychology, 22,* 453–474.

Albert, E. A., Warner, D. L., Hatcher, R. A., Trussell, J., & Bennett, C. (1995). Condom use among female commercial sex workers in Nevada's legal brothels. *American Journal of Public Health, 85,* 1514–1520.

Allen, S., Serufilira, A., Bogaerts, J., Van de Perre, P., Nsengumuremyi, F., Lindan, C., Carael, M., Wolf, W., Coates, T., & Hulley, S. (1992). Confidential HIV testing and condom promotion in Africa: Impact on HIV and gonorrhea rates. *JAMA, 268,* 3338–3343.

Allen, S., Tice, J., Van de Perre, P., Serufilira, A., Hudes, E., Nsengumuremyi, F., Bogaerts, J., Lindan, C., & Hulley, S. (1992). Effect of serotesting with counselling on condom use and seroconversion among HIV discordant couples in Africa. *British Medical Journal, 304,* 1605–1609.

Altman, D. (1994). *Power and community: Organizational and cultural responses to AIDS.* London, England: Taylor & Francis.

Altman, D. A. (1995). Sustaining interventions in community systems: On the relationship between researchers and communities. *Health Psychology, 14,* 526–536.

Amaro, H. (1995). Love, sex, and power. Considering women's realities in HIV prevention. *American Psychologist, 50,* 437–447.

Analysis of Sexual Behaviour in France. (1992). A comparison between two modes of investigation: Telephone survey and face-to-face survey. *AIDS, 6,* 315–323.

Anderson, J. E., Cheney, R., Faruque, S., Long, A., Toomey, K., & Wiebel, W. (1996). Stages of change for HIV risk behavior: Injecting drug users in five cities. *Drugs & Society, 9,* 1–17.

Apt, C., & Hurlbert, F. (1992). The female sensation seeker and marital sexuality. *Journal of Sex and Marital Therapy, 18,* 315–324.

Aral, S. O. (1993). Heterosexual transmission of HIV: The role of other sexually transmitted infections and behavior in its epidemiology, prevention and control. *Annual Review of Public Health, 14,* 451–467.

178

Aral, S. O., & Holmes, K. K. (1991). Sexually transmitted diseases in the AIDS era. *Scientific American, 264,* 62–69.

Aral, S. O., & Peterman, T. (1996). Measuring outcomes of behavioural interventions for STD/HIV prevention. *International Journal of STD & AIDS, 7* (Suppl. 2), 30–38.

Aral, S. O., & Wasserheit, J. N. (1995). Interactions among HIV, other sexually transmitted diseases, socioeconomic status, and poverty in women. In A. O'Leary & L. S. Jemmott (Eds.), *Women at risk: Issues in the primary prevention of AIDS* (pp. 13–41). New York: Plenum.

Auerbach, J. D., Wypijewska, C., & Brodie, H. K. (1994). *AIDS and behavior: An integrated approach.* Washington, DC: National Academy Press.

Ayeunie, S., Groves, R., Bruzzese, A. M., Ruprecht, R., Kupper, T., & Langhoff, E. (1995). Acutely infected Langerhans cells are more efficient than T cells in disseminating HIV type 1 activated T cells following a short cell-cell contact. *AIDS Research and Human Retroviruses, 11,* 877–884.

Baba, T. W., Trichel, A. M., An, L., Liska, V., Martin, L., Murphey–Corb, M., & Ruprecht, R. M. (1996). Infection and AIDS in adult macaques after nontraumatic oral exposure of cell-free SIV. *Science, 272,* 1486–1489.

Baier, J. L., Rosenzweig, M. G., & Whipple, E. G. (1991). Patterns of sexual behavior, coercion, and victimization of university students. *Journal of College Student Development, 32,* 310–322.

Baker, A., & Dixon, J. (1991). Motivational interviewing for HIV risk reduction. In W. R. Miller & S. Rollnick (Eds.), *Motivational interviewing: Preparing people for change* (pp. 293–302). New York: Guilford.

Baker, A., Heather, N., Wodak, A., Dixon, J., & Holt, P. (1993). Evaluation of a cognitive-behavioural intervention for HIV prevention among injecting drug users. *AIDS, 7,* 247–256.

Baker, A., Kochan, N., Dixon, J., Wodak, A., & Heather, N. (1994). HIV risk-taking behavior among injection drug users not currently in treatment. *Drug and Alcohol Dependence, 34,* 155–160.

Bandura, A. (1986). *Social foundations of thought and action: A social cognitive theory.* Englewood Cliffs, NJ: Prentice–Hall.

Bandura, A. (1989). Perceived self-efficacy in the exercise of control over AIDS infection. In V. M. Mays, G. W. Albee, & S. F. Schneider (Eds.), *Primary prevention of AIDS: Psychological approaches* (pp. 128–141). Newbury Park, CA: Sage.

Bandura, A. (1994). Social cognitive theory and exercise of control over HIV infection. In R. DiClemente & J. Peterson (Eds.), *Preventing AIDS: Theories, methods, and behavioral interventions* (pp. 25–60). New York: Plenum.

Bandura, A. (1997). *Self-efficacy: The exercise of control.* New York: Freeman.

Baron, P., & Watters, R. G. (1981). Effects of goal-setting and of goal levels on weight loss induced by self-monitoring of caloric intake. *Canadian Journal of Behavioural Science, 13,* 161–170.

Barth, R. J., & Kinder, B. N. (1987). The mislabeling of sexual impulsivity. *Journal of Sex & Marital Therapy, 13,* 15–23.

Bartlett, J. G. (1993). *The Johns Hopkins Hospital guide to medical care of patients with HIV infection,* (3rd ed.). Baltimore: Williams & Wilkins.

Bayer, R., Stryker, J., & Smith, M. D. (1995). Testing for HIV infection at home. *The New England Journal of Medicine, 332,* 1296–1299.

Bayer, R., & Toomey, K. E. (1992). Health law and ethics: HIV prevention and the two faces of partner notification. *American Journal of Public Health, 82,* 1153–1164.

Beck, E. J., Mandalia, S., Leonard, K., Griffith, R. J., Harris, J., & Miller, D. (1996). Case-control study of sexually transmitted diseases as cofactors for HIV-1 transmission. *International Journal of STD & AIDS, 7,* 34–38.

Belcher, L., Kalichman, S. C., Topping, M., Smith, S., Emshoff, J., Norris, F., & Nurss, J. (1997). *A randomized trial of a brief HIV risk reduction counseling intervention for women.* Manuscript submitted for publication.

Benjamin, J., Li, L., Patterson, C., Greenberg, B., Murphy, D., & Hamer, D. (1996). Population and familial association between D4 dopamine receptor gene and measures of novelty seeking. *Nature Genetics, 12,* 81–84.

Bergey, E., Cho, M., Blumberg, B., Hammarskjold, M. L., Rekosh, D., Epstein, L., & Levine, M. (1994). Interaction of HIV-1 and human salivary mucins. *Journal of Acquired Immune Deficiency Syndromes, 1,* 995–1002.

Bergey, E. J., Cho, M. I., Hammarskjold, M. L., Rekosh, D., Levine, M. J., Blumberg, B. M., & Epstein, L. G. (1993). Aggregation of human immunodeficiency virus type 1 by human salivary secretions. *Critical Review of Oral Biological Medicine, 4,* 467–474.

Beutler, L., Williams, R., Wakefield, P., & Entwistle, S. (1995). Bridging scientist and practitioner perspectives in clinical psychology. *American Psychologist, 50,* 984–994.

Bevier, P., Chiasson, M., Heffernan, R., & Castro, K. (1995). Women at a sexually transmitted disease clinic who report same-sex contact: Their HIV seroprevalence and risk behaviors. *American Journal of Public Health, 85,* 1366–1371.

Biddle, N., Conte, L., & Diamond, E. (1993). AIDS in the media: Entertainment or infotainment. In S. C. Ratzan (Ed.), *AIDS: Effective health communication for the 90s* (pp. 141–150). Washington, DC: Taylor & Francis.

Billy, J. O. G., Tranfer, K., Grady, W., & Klepinger, D. H. (1993). The sexual behavior of men in the United States. *Family Planning Perspectives, 25,* 52–60.

Blakely, C. H., Mayer, J. P., Gottschalk, R. G., Schmitt, N., Davidson, W. S., Roitman, D. B., & Emshoff, J. G. (1987). The fidelity-adaptation debate: Implications for the implementation of public sector social programs. *American Journal of Community Psychology, 15,* 253–268.

Blendon, R. J., Heimendinger, J., & Marwick, C. (1994). Workshop D: NIH interface with public translation policy. *Preventive Medicine, 23,* 556–557.

Boast, N., & Coid, J. (1994). Homosexual erotomania and HIV infection. *British Journal of Psychiatry, 164,* 842–846.

Boekeloo, B., Schiavo, L., Rabin, D. L., Conlon, R. T., Jordan, C. S., & Mundt, D. J. (1994). Self-reports of HIV risk factors by patients at a sexually transmitted disease clinic: Audio vs. written questionnaires. *American Journal of Public Health, 84,* 754–760.

Booth, R. E., Watters, J. K., & Chitwood, D. D. (1993). HIV risk-related sex behaviors among injection drug users, crack smokers, and injection drug users who smoke crack. *American Journal of Public Health, 83,* 1144–1148.

Booth, W. (1988). AIDS and drug abuse: No quick fix. *Science, 239,* 717–719.

Borelli, B., & Mermelstein, R. (1994). Goal setting and behavior change in a smoking cessation program. *Cognitive Therapy and Research, 18,* 69–83.

Bradburn, N., & Sudman, S. (1979). *Improving interview method and questionnaire design.* San Francisco: Jossey-Bass.

Brammer, L. (1973). *The helping relationship: Process and skills.* Englewood Cliffs, NJ: Prentice-Hall.

Branson, B. M., Ransom, R., Peterman, T., & Zaidi, A. (1996). *Randomized control trial of intensive group counseling to reduce risk behaviors in high-risk STD clinic patients.* Paper presented at the meeting of the International AIDS Conference, Vancouver, Canada.

Broadhead, R. S., & Fox, K. J. (1990). Takin' it to the streets: AIDS outreach as ethnography. *Journal of Contemporary Ethnography, 19,* 322–348.

Brody, S. (1995a). Heterosexual transmission of HIV. *New England Journal of Medicine, 331,* 1718.

Brody, S. (1995b). Patients misrepresenting their risk factors for AIDS. *International Journal of STD & AIDS, 6,* 392–398.

Brown, B. S. (1995). Reducing impediments to technology transfer in drug abuse programming. In T. E. Backer, S. L. David, & G. Soucy (Eds.), *Reviewing the behavioral science knowledge base on technology transfer* (pp. 169–185). Rockville, MD: National Institute on Drug Abuse.

Brown, L. K., & Fritz, G. K. (1988). AIDS education in the schools: A literature review as a guide for curriculum planning. *Clinical Pediatrics, 27*, 311–316.

Brown, L. K., Fritz, G. K., & Barone, V. J. (1989). The impact of AIDS education on junior and senior high school students. *Journal of Adolescent Health Care, 10*, 386–392.

Brownell, K. D., Marlatt, G. A., Lichtenstein, E., & Wilson, G. T. (1986). Understanding and preventing relapse. *American Psychologist, 41*, 765–782.

Bryan, A. D., Aiken, L. S., & West, S. G. (1996). Increasing condom use: Evaluation of a theory-based intervention to prevent sexually transmitted diseases in young women. *Health Psychology, 15*, 371–382.

Caceres, C. F., van Griensven, G. (1994). Male homosexual transmission of HIV-1. *AIDS, 8*, 1051–1061.

Calsyn, D. A., Saxon, A., Freeman, G., & Whittaker, S. (1992). Ineffectiveness of AIDS education and HIV antibody testing in reducing high-risk behaviors among injection drug users. *American Journal of Public Health, 82*, 573–575.

Cambell, C.A. (1990). Prostitution and AIDS. In D.G. Ostrow (Ed.), *Behavioral aspects of AIDS*. New York: Plenum.

Carballo-Dieguez, A., Remien, R., Dolezal, C., & Wagner, G. (1997). Unsafe sex in the primary relationships of Puerto Rican men who have sex with men. *AIDS & Behavior, 1*, 9–17.

Card, J. J., Niego, S., Mallari, A., & Farrell, W. S. (1996). The program archive on sexuality, health & adolescence: Promising "prevention programs in a box". *Family Planning Perspectives, 28*, 210–220.

Carey, M. P., Maisto, S. A., Kalichman, S. C., Forsyth, A., Wright, I., & Johnson, B. T. (1997). Enhancing motivation to reduce risk for HIV infection for economically disadvantaged urban women. *Journal of Consulting and Clinical Psychology, 65*, 531–541.

Carey, R. F., Herman, W. A., Retta, S. M., Rinaldi, J. E., Herman, B. A., & Athey, T. W. (1992). Effectiveness of latex condoms as a barrier to human immunodeficiency virus-sized particles under conditions of simulated use. *Sexually Transmitted Diseases, 19*, 230–233.

Catania, J. A., Coates, T. J., Stall, R., Turner, H., Peterson, J., Hearst, N., Dolcini, M. M., Hudes, E., Gagnon, J., Wiley, J., & Groves, R. (1992). Prevalence of AIDS-related risk factors and condom use in the United States. *Science, 258*, 1101–1106.

Catania, J. A., Gibson, D., Marin, B., Coates, T., & Greenblatt, R. (1990). Response bias in assessing sexual behaviors relevant to HIV transmission. *Evaluation and Program Planning, 13*, 19–29.

Catania, J. A., Gibson, D., Chitwood, D., & Coates, T. J. (1990). Methodological problems in AIDS behavioral research: Influences on measurement error and participation bias in studies of sexual behavior. *Psychological Bulletin, 108*, 339–362.

Catania, J. A., Kegeles, S. M., & Coates, T. J. (1990). Towards an understanding of risk behavior: An AIDS risk reduction model (ARRM). *Health Education Quarterly, 17*, 53–72.

Cates, W., Toomey, K., Havlak, G. R., Bowen, G., & Hinman, A. (1990). Partner notification and confidentiality of the index patient: Its role in preventing HIV. *Sexually Transmitted Diseases, 19*, 113–114.

CDC. (1981a). Kaposi's sarcoma and *Pneumocystis pneumonia* among homosexual men—New York City and California. *Morbidity and Mortality Weekly Report, 30*, 305–308.

CDC. (1981b). *Pneumocystis* pneumonia- Los Angeles. *Morbidity and Mortality Weekly Report, 30*, 250–252.

CDC. (1988). *Guide to public health practice: HIV partner notification strategies.* Washington, DC: Public Health Foundation.

CDC. (1992). Condom use among male injecting-drug users—New York City, 1987–1990. *Morbidity and Mortality Weekly Report, 41*, 617–620.

CDC. (1993). Condoms and their use in preventing HIV infection and other STDs. *CDC Newsletter.* Atlanta: Author.

CDC. (1995b). Case-control study of HIV seroconversion in health case workers after percutaneous exposures to HIV infected blood—France, United Kingdom, and United States, January 1988–August 1994. *Morbidity and Mortality Weekly Report, 44*, 929–933.

CDC. (1996). Continued sexual risk behavior among HIV seropositive, drug using men—Atlanta; Washington, DC; and San Juan, Puerto Rico, 1993. *Morbidity and Mortality Weekly Report, 45*, 150–152.

CDC. (1997). *HIV/AIDS surveillance report: Midyear edition.* Atlanta, GA: Author.

Chapman, S., Stoker, L., Ward, M., Porritt, D., & Fahey, P. (1990). Discriminant attitudes and beliefs about condoms in young, multi-partner heterosexuals. *International Journal of STD and AIDS, 1*, 422–428.

Chavis, D. M., Stucky, P., & Wandersman, A. (1983). Returning basic research to the community: A relationship between scientists and citizen. *American Psychologist, 38*, 424–434.

Chiasson, M. A., Stonebruner, R., & Joseph, S. (1990). Human immunodeficiency virus transmission through artificial insemination. *Journal of Acquired Immune Deficiency Syndromes, 3*, 69–72.

Chaisson, R. E., Moss, R. A., Onishi, R., Osmond, D., & Carlson, J. R. (1987). Human immunodeficiency virus infection in heterosexual intravenous drug users in San Francisco. *American Journal of Public Health, 77*, 169–171.

Choi, K–H., Lew, S., Vittinghoff, E., Catania, J. A., Barrett, D. C., & Coates, T. J. (1996). The efficacy of brief group counseling in HIV risk reduction among homosexual Asian and Pacific Islander men. *AIDS, 10*, 81–87.

Choi, K–H., Rickman, R., & Catania, J. A. (1994). What heterosexual adults believe about condoms. *The New England Journal of Medicine, 331*, 406–407.

Chorba, T. L., Holman, R. C., & Evatt, B. L. (1993). Heterosexual and mother-to-child transmission of AIDS in the hemophilia community. *Public Health Reports, 108*, 99–105.

Christopher, F. S., & Roosa, M. W. (1990). An evaluation of an adolescent pregnancy prevention program: Is "just say no" enough? *Family Relations, 39*, 68–72.

Chu, S. Y., Conti, L., Schable, B., & Diaz, T. (1994). Female-to-female sexual contact and HIV transmission. *JAMA, 272*, 443.

Cleary, P. D., von Devanter, N., Rogers, T., Singer, E., Shipton–Levy, R., Steilen, M., Stuart, A., Avorn, J., & Pindyck, J. (1991). Behavior changes after notification of HIV infection. *American Journal of Public Health, 81*, 1586–1590.

Clift, A., Wilkins, J., & Davidson, A. (1993). Impulsiveness, venturesomeness, and sexual risk taking among heterosexual gum clinic attendees. *Personality and Individual Differences, 15*, 403–410.

Coates, R., Soskolne, C., Calzavara, L., Read, S., Fanning, N., Shephard, F., Klein, M., & Johnson, J. (1986). The reliability of sexual histories in AIDS related research: Evaluation of an interview administered questionnaire. *Canadian Journal of Public Health, 77*, 343–348.

Coates, T. J., Agleton, P., Gutzwiller, F., Des Jarlais, D., Kihara, M., Kippax, S., Schechter, M., & van den Hoek, J. (1996). HIV prevention in developed countries. *Lancet, 348*, 1143–1148.

Coates, T. J., Stall, R. D., Kegeles, S. M., Lo, B., Morin, S. F., & McKusick, L. (1988). AIDS antibody testing. Will it stop the AIDS epidemic? Will it help people infected with HIV? *American Psychologists, 43*, 859–864.

Cochran, S., & Mays, V. (1990). Sex, lies, and HIV. *New England Journal of Medicine, 322*, 774–775.

Cohen, H., Marmor, M., Wolfe, H., & Ribble, D. (1993) Risk assessment of HIV transmission among lesbians. *Journal of Acquired Immune Deficiency Syndromes and Human Retrovirology, 6*, 1173–1174.

Cohen, J. (1997). Advances painted in shades of gray at a D. C. conference. *Science, 275*, 615–616.

Cohen, S., & Williamson, G. (1991). Stress and infectious disease in humans. *Psychological Bulletin, 109*, 5–24.

Collins, C., & Franks, P. (1996). Improving the use of behavioral research in the CDC's HIV prevention community planning process. *Monograph series of Marketing HIV Prevention.* (Occasional paper #1).

Colón, H. M., Sahai, H., Robles, R. R., & Matos, T. D. (1995). Effects of a community outreach program in HIV risk behaviors among injection drug users in San Juan Puerto Rico: An analysis of trends. *AIDS Education and Prevention, 7,* 195–209.

Conant, M., Hardy, D., Sernatinger, J., Spicer, D., & Levy, J. A. (1986). Condoms prevent transmission of AIDS-associated retrovirus. *JAMA, 255,* 1706.

Consumer Reports. (1995, May). How reliable are condoms? *Consumer Reports,* 320–325.

Cooper, D. A. (1994). Early antiretroviral therapy. *AIDS, 8,* S9–S14.

Corby, N. H., Enguídanos, S. M., & Kay, L. S. (1996). Development and use of role model stories in a community level HIV risk reduction intervention. *Public Health Reports, 111,* (Suppl. 1), 54–58.

Corby, N. H. & Wolitski, R. (1997). *Community HIV prevention: The Long Beach AIDS Community Demonstration Project.* Long Beach: University of California Press.

Coyle, K., Kirby, D., Parcel, G., Basen–Engquist, K., Banspach, S., Rugg, D., & Weil, M. (1996). Safer choices: A multicomponent school-based HIV/STD and pregnancy prevention program for adolescents. *Journal of School Health, 66,* 89–94.

Crawford, I., & Jason, L. A. (1990). Strategies for implementing a media-based AIDS prevention program. *Professional Psychology: Research and Practice, 21,* 219–221.

Crawford, I., Jason, L. A., Riordan, N., Kaufman, J., Salina, D., Sawalski, L., Ho, F. C., & Zolik, E. (1990). A multimedia-based approach to increasing communication and the level of AIDS knowledge within families. *Journal of Community Psychology, 18,* 361–373.

Darrow, W. W., Echenberg, D. F., Jaffe, H. W., O'Malley, P. M., Byers, R. H., Getchell, J. P., & Curran, J. W. (1987). Risk factors for human immunodeficiency virus (HIV) infections in homosexual men. *American Journal of Public Health, 77,* 479–483.

Davidson, S., Dew, M. A., Penkower, L., Becker, J., Kingsley, L., & Sullivan, P. (1995). Substance use and sexual behavior among homosexual men at risk for HIV infection: Psychosocial mediators. *Psychology and Health, 7,* 259–272.

Dean, L., & Meyer, I. (1995). HIV prevalence and sexual behavior in a cohort of New York City gay men (aged 18–24). *Journal of Acquired Immune Deficiency Syndromes and Human Retrovirology, 8,* 208–211.

Deeks, S. G., Smith, M., Holodnly, M., & Kahn, J. (1997). HIV-1 protease inhibitors: A review for clinicians. *JAMA, 277,* 145–153.

Deren, S., Davis, W. R., Beardsley, M., Tortu, S., & Clatts, M. (1995). Outcomes of a risk-reduction intervention with high-risk populations: The Harlem AIDS projects. *AIDS Education and Prevention, 7(5),* 379–390.

Deren, S., Stephens, R., Davis, W. R., Feucht, T., & Tortu, S. (1994). The impact of providing incentives for attendance at AIDS prevention sessions. *Public Health Reports, 109,* 548–554.

Des Jarlais, D. C., Abdul–Quader, A., Minkoff, H. (1991).Crack use and multiple AIDS risk behaviors. *Journal of Acquired Immune Deficiency Syndromes, 4,* 446–447.

Detels, R., English, P., & Vischer, B. R. (1989). Seroconversion, sexual activity and condom use among HIV seronegative men followed for up to 2 years. *Journal of Acquired Immune Deficiency Syndromes, 2,* 77–83.

De Vincenzi, I. (1994). A longitudinal study of human immunodeficiency virus transmission by heterosexual partners. *New England Journal of Medicine, 331,* 341–346.

De Wit, J. (1994). *Prevention of HIV infection among homosexual men: Behavior change and behavioral determinants.* Amsterdam: Thesis Publishers.

De Wit, J. (1996, July). *The epidemic of HIV among young gay men.* XI International Conference on AIDS, Vancouver.

Diaz, T., Chu, S. Y., Conti, L., Sorvillo, F., Checko, P. J., Hermann, P., Fann, A. S., Frederick, M., Boyd, D., Mokotoff, E., Rietmeijer, C. A., Herr, M., & Samuel, M. C. (1994). Risk behaviors of persons with heterosexually acquired HIV infection in the

United States: Results of a multistate surveillance project. *Journal of Acquired Immune Deficiency Syndromes, 7*, 958–963.

DiClemente, R. J., Durbin, M., Siegel, D., Krasnovsky, F., Lazarus, N., & Comacho, T. (1992). Determinants of condom use among junior high school students in a minority, inner-city school district. *Pediatrics, 89*, 197–202.

DiClemente, R., & Wingood, G. (1995). A randomized controlled trial of an HIV sexual risk-reduction intervention for young African-American women. *JAMA, 274,* 1271–1276.

DiFranceisco, W., Ostrow, D., & Chmiel, J. (1996). Sexual adventurism, high-risk behavior, and human immunodeficiency virus-1 seroconversion among the Chicago MACS-CCS Cohort, 1984–1992: A case-control study. *Sexually Transmitted Diseases, 23*, 453–460.

DiIorio, C., Parsons, M., Lehr, S., Adame, D., & Carlone, J. (1993). Factors associated with use of safer sex practices among college freshmen. *Research in Nursing and Health, 16*, 343–350.

Dilley, J. W., Woods, W. J., & McFarland, W. (1997). Are advances in treatment changing views about high-risk sex? *New England Journal of Medicine, 337*, 501–502.

Direct Access. (1996). *The Confide Home Test Kit.* Direct Access, Inc.

Doll, L. S., Harrison, J., Frey, R., McKirnan, D., Bartholow, B., Douglas, J., Joy, D., Blan, G., & Doetsch, J. (1994). Failure to disclose HIV risk among gay and bisexual men attending sexually transmitted disease clinics. *American Journal of Preventive Medicine, 10*, 125–129.

Doll, L. S., & Kennedy, M. B. (1994). HIV counseling and testing: What is it and how well does it work? In S. Schochetman & J. R. George (Eds.), *AIDS testing: A comprehensive guide to technical, medical, social, legal, and management issues* (2nd ed.), (pp. 302–319). New York: Springer–Verlag.

Downey, L., Ryan, R., Roffman, R., & Kulich, M. (1995). How could I forget? Inaccurate memories of sexually intimate moments. *Journal of Sex Research, 32*, 177–191.

Downs, A. M., & De Vincenzi, I. (1996). Probability of heterosexual transmission of HIV: Relationships to the number of unprotected sexual contacts. *Journal of Acquired Immune Deficiency Syndromes and Human Retrovirology, 11*, 388–395.

Dubbert, P. M., & Wilson, G. T. (1984). Goal-setting and spouse involvement in the treatment of obesity. *Behavioral Research and Therapy, 22*, 227–242.

Duesberg, P. (1988). HIV is not the cause of AIDS. *Science, 241*, 514, 517.

Duesberg, P. H. (1989). Human immunodeficiency virus and acquired immunodeficiency syndrome: Correlation but not causation. *Proceedings of the National Academy of Science, 86*, 755–764.

Durlak, J. A. (1979). Comparative effectiveness of paraprofessional and professional helpers. *Psychological Bulletin, 86*, 80–92.

D'Zurilla, T. J., & Goldfried, M. R. (1971). Problem solving and behavior modification. *Journal of Abnormal Psychology, 78*, 107–126.

Ebstein, R., Novick, O., Umansky, R., Priel, B., Osher, Y., Blaine, D., Bennett, E., Nemanov, L., Katz, M., & Belmaker, R. (1996). Dopamine D4 receptor (D4DR) exon III polymorphism associated with the human personality trait for novelty seeking. *Nature Genetics, 12*, 78–80.

Edwards, S. K., & White, C. (1995). HIV seroconversion illness after orogenital contact with successful contact tracing. *International Journal of STD & AIDS, 6*, 50–51.

Egan, G. (1982). *The skilled helper: Model, skills, and methods for effective helping* (2nd ed.). Monterey, CA: Brooks/Cole Publishing Company.

El-Bassel, N., & Schilling, R. F. (1991). Drug use and sexual behavior of indigent African American men. *Public Health Reports, 106*, 586–590.

Eldin, B., Irwin, K., Faraque, S., McCoy, C., Word, C., Serrano, Y., Inciardi, J., Bowser, B., Schilling, R., & Holmberg, S. (1994). Intersecting epidemic—crack cocaine use and HIV infection among inner-city young adults. *New England Journal of Medicine, 331*, 422–427.

Ericksen, K. P., & Trocki, K. F. (1992). Behavioral risk factors for sexually transmitted diseases in American households. *Social Science Medicine, 34*, 843–853.

Essex, M. (1995). The HIV-1 vaccine dilemma: Lessons from the cat. *Journal of NIH Research, 7,* 37–42.

Exner, T. M., Meyer–Bahlburg, H. F. L., & Ehrhardt, A. A. (1992). Sexual self control as a mediator of high risk sexual behavior in a New York City cohort of HIV+ and HIV-gay men. *The Journal of Sex Research, 29,* 389–406.

Fabj, V., & Sobnosky, M. J. (1993). Responses from the street ACT UP and community organizing against AIDS. In S. C. Ratzan (Ed.), *AIDS: Effective health communication for the 90s* (pp. 91–109). Washington, DC: Taylor & Francis.

Farr, G., Gabelnick, H., Sturgen, K., & Dorflinger, L. (1994). Contraceptive efficacy and acceptability of the female condom. *American Journal of Public Health, 84,* 1960–1964.

Feldblum, P. J., & Fortney, J. A. (1988). Condoms, spermicides and the transmission of human immunodeficieny virus. *American Journal of Public Health, 78,* 52–54.

Fishbein, M. (1996). Editorial: Great expectations, or do we ask too much from community-level interventions? *American Journal of Public Health, 86,* 1075–1076.

Fishbein, M., & Ajzen, I. (1975). *Belief, attitude, intention, & behavior: An introduction to theory and research.* Reading, MA: Addison Wesley.

Fishbein, M., Middlestadt, S., & Hitchcock, P. (1994). Using information to change sexually transmitted disease-related behaviors: An analysis based on theory of reasoned action. In R. DiClemente & J. Peterson (Eds.), *Preventing AIDS: Theories, methods, and behavioral interventions* (pp. 61–77). New York: Plenum.

Fishbein, M., & Rhodes, F. (1997). Using behavioral theory in HIV prevention. In N. Corby & R. Wolitski (Eds.), *Community HIV prevention: The Long Beach AIDS community demonstration project* (pp. 21–30). Long Beach,: University of California Press.

Fisher, J. D., & Fisher, W. A. (1992). Changing AIDS-risk behavior. *Psychological Bulletin, 111,* 455–474.

Fisher, J. D., & Misovich, S. J. (1990). Social influence and AIDS-preventive behavior. In J. Edwards, R. S. Tindale, L. Heath, & E. J. Posavac (Eds.), *Social Influence Processes and Prevention* (pp. 39–70). New York: Plenum.

Folkman, S., Chesney, M., Pollack, L., & Phillips, C. (1992). Stress, coping, and high-risk sexual behavior, *Health Psychology, 11,* 218–222.

Fordyce, E. J., Williams, R. D., Surick, I. W., Shum, R., Quintyne, R., & Thomas, P. (1995). Trends in the AIDS epidemic among men who reported sex with men in New York City: 1981–1993. *AIDS Education and Prevention, 7,* 3–13.

Forsyth, A. D., Carey, M. P., & Fuqua, W. (1997). Evaluation of the validity of the condom use self-efficacy scale (CUSES) in young men using two behavioral simulations. *Health Psychology, 16,* 175–178.

Fox, P., Wolff, A., Yeh, C., Atkinson, J., & Baum, B. (1989). Salivary inhibition of HIV-1 infectivity: Functional properties and distribution in men, women, and children. *Journal of the American Dental Association, 118,* 709–711.

Fox, R., Odaka, N., Brookmeyer, R., & Polk, B. F. (1987). Effect of HIV antibody disclosure on subsequent sexual activity in homosexual men. *AIDS, 1,* 241–246.

Friedman, S., Des Jarlais, D., & Ward, T. (1994). Social models for changing health-relevant behavior. In R. Di Clemente & J. Peterson (Eds.), *Preventing AIDS: Theories, methods, and behavioral interventions* (pp. 95–116). New York: Plenum.

Frutchey, C., Blankenship, W., Stall, R., & Henne, J. (1995). *Ability to envision a future predicts safe sex among gay men.* Unpublished manuscript.

Fujita, B. N., Wagner, N. N., Perthou, N., & Pion, R. J. (1971). The effects of an interview on attitudes and behavior. *Journal of Sex Research, 7,* 138–152.

Fullilove, R. E., Fullilove, M. T., Haynes, K., & Gross, S. A. (1990). Black women and AIDS prevention: A view towards understanding the gender rules. *Journal of Sex Research, 27,* 47–64.

Fultz, P. N. (1986). Components of saliva inactivate human immunodeficiency virus. *Lancet, ii,* 345–349.

Gay and Lesbian Medical Association. (1996, Spring). GLMA Position on male-to-male oral-genital sex. *GLMA Newsletter,* p. 22.

Gay Men's Health Crisis. (1995). *House of latex project: Volunteer liaison training curriculum.* New York City: Author.

Gayle, H. D., & D'Angelo, L. J. (1991). Epidemiology of acquired immunodeficiency syndrome and human immunodeficiency virus infection in adolescents. *Pediatric Infectious Disease Journal, 10,* 322–328.

Gendin, S. (1997). Riding bareback: Skin-on-skin sex—been there, done that, want more. *Poz Magazine,* June, 64–65.

Gerber, A. R., Valdiserri, R. O., Holtgrave, D. R., Jones, S., West, G. R., Hinman, A. R., & Curran, J. W. (1993). Preventive services guidelines for primary care clinicians caring for adults and adolescents infected with the Human Immunodeficiency Virus. *Archives of Family Medicine, 2,* 969–979.

Gerberding, J. L. (1997). Limiting the risks of health care workers. In M. A. Sande, & P. A. Volberding (Eds.), *The Medical Management of AIDS* (pp. 75–85). Philadelphia: W. B. Saunders.

Gibson, D. R., Wermuth, L., Lovelle–Drache, J., Ham, J., & Sorenson, J. L. (1989). Brief counselling to reduce AIDS risk in intravenous drug users and their sexual partners: Preliminary results. *Counselling Psychology Quarterly, 2,* 15–19.

Gidycz, C. A., & Koss, M. P. (1989). The impact of adolescent sexual victimization: Standardized measures of anxiety, depression, and behavioral deviancy. *Violence and Victims, 4,* 139–149.

Glasner, P. D., & Kaslow, R. A. (1990). The epidemiology of human immunodeficiency virus infection. *Journal of Consulting and Clinical Psychology, 58,* 13–21.

Gold, R. S., & Skinner, M. (1992). Situational factors and thought processes associated with unprotected intercourse in young gay men. *AIDS, 6,* 1021–1030.

Gold, R. S., & Skinner, M. (1994). Unprotected anal intercourse in HIV infected and non-infected gay men. *Journal of Sex Research, 31,* 59–77.

Goldstein, E., Wrubel, J., Faigeles, B., & DeCarlo, P. (1996). *Do researchers reach non-governmental organizations in the United Sates?* XI International Conference on AIDS, Vancouver.

Gollub, E. L., & Stein, Z. A. (1993). Commentary: The new female condom- item 1 on a women's AIDS prevention agenda. *American Journal of Public Health, 83,* 498–500.

Golombok, S., Sketchley, J., & Rust, J. (1989). Condom failure among homosexual men. *Journal of Acquired Immune Deficiency Syndromes, 2,* 404–409.

Gordon, C., Forsyth, A., Weinhardt, L., & Carey, M. P. (1995). Assessment of behavioral skills in sexual health research. *The Health Psychologist, 17,* 6–7, 14.

Grady, C. (1995). *The search for an AIDS Vaccine: Ethical issues in the development and testing of a preventive HIV vaccine.* Bloomington: Indiana University Press.

Grady, W. R., Klepinger, D. H., Billy, J. O., & Tanfer, K. (1993). Condom characteristics: The perspectives and preferences of men in the United States. *Family Planning Perspectives, 25,* 67–73.

Grant, D., & Anns, M. (1988). Counseling AIDS antibody-positive clients: reactions and treatment. *American Psychologist, 18,* 72–74.

Greenberg, J., MacGowan, R., Long, A., Fernando, D., Cheney, R., Sterk, C., & Wiebel, W. (1997). *Does street outreach affect use of medical services by injecting drug users?* Unpublished manuscript.

Grimley, D. M., Prochaska, G. E., & Prochaska, J. O. (1993). Condom use assertiveness and the stages of change with main and other partners. *Journal of Applied Biobehavioral Research, 1*(2), 152–173.

Grinstead, O. A., Peterson, J. L., Faigeles, B., & Catania, J. (1997). Antibody testing and condom use among heterosexual African-Americans at risk for HIV infection: The National AIDS Behavioral Surveys. *American Journal of Public Health, 87,* 857–859.

Grosskurth, H., Mosha, F., Todd, J., Mwjarubi, E., Klokke, A., Mayaud, P., Changalucha, J., Nicoll, A., Ka–Gina, G., Newell, J., Mugeye, K., Mabey, D., & Hayes, R. (1995). Impact of improved treatment of sexually transmitted diseases on HIV infection in rural Tanzania: Randomised controlled trial. *Lancet, 346,* 530–536.

Grunseit, A. C., Rodden, P., Crawford, J., & Kippax, S. (1994). Patterns of serologic testing in HIV-1 seronegative men. *Annual Conference Australia's HIV Medicine, 6,* 16.

Guenther–Grey, C. A., Johnson, W. D., Higgins, D. L., Fishbein, M., & Moseley, R. R. (1996). Community-level prevention of human immunodeficiency virus infection among high risk populations: The AIDS Community Demonstrations Projects. *Morbidity and Mortality Weekly Report, 45,* (RR–6).

Guttmacher, S., Lieberman, L., Ward, D., Freudenberg, N., Radosh, A., & Des Jarlais, D. (1997). Condom availability in New York City public high schools: Relationships to condom use and sexual behavior. *American Journal of Public Health, 87,* 1427–1433.

Haffner, D. W., & Mayer, R. (1997). Sexuality educator's perspective. *AIDS and Behavior, 1,* 208–209.

Halpern, C. T., Udry, J. R., & Suchindran, C. (1994). Effects of repeated questionnaire administration in longitudinal studies of adolescent males' sexual behavior. *Archives of Sexual Behavior, 23,* 41–57.

Hammer, S. M., Katzenstein, D. A., Hughes, M. D., Gundacker, H., Scholley, R. T., Haubrich, R. H., Henry, K., Lederman, M. M., Phair, J. P., Niu, M., Hirsch, M. S., & Merigan, T. C. (1996). A trial comparing nucleoside monotherapy with combination therapy in HIV-infected adults with CD4 cell counts from 200–500 per cubic millimeter. *New England Journal of Medicine, 335,* 1081–1090.

Hatcher, R. A., & Hughes, M. (1988). The truth about condoms. *SIECUS Report, 17,* 1–9.

Haverkos, H. W., & Battjes, R. J. (1992). Female-to-male transmission of HIV. *JAMA, 268,* 1855–1856.

Heckman, T., Kelly, J., Sikkema, K., Cargill, V., Norman, A., Fuqua, W., Wagstaff, D., Solomon, L., Roffman, R., Crumble, D., Perry, M., Winett, R., Anderson, E., Mercer, M., & Hoffman, R. (1995). HIV risk characteristics of young adult, adult, and older adult women who live in inner-city housing developments: Implications for prevention. *Journal of Women's Health, 4,* 397–406.

Hein, K. (1990). Lessons from New York City on HIV/AIDS in adolescents. *New York State Journal of Medicine, 90,* 143–145.

Higgins, D. L., Galavotti, C., O'Reilly, K. R., Schnell, D. J., Moore, M., Rugg, D. L., & Johnson, R. (1991). Evidence for the effects of HIV antibody counseling and testing on risk behavior. *JAMA, 266,* 2419–2429.

Ho, D. D. (1995). Time to hit HIV, early and hard. *New England Journal of Medicine, 333,* 450–451.

Ho, D. D. (1996). Therapy of HIV infections: Problems and prospects. *Bulletin of the New York Academy of Medicine, 73,* 37–45.

Hobfoll, S. E., (1989). Conservation of resources: A new attempt at conceptualizing stress. *American Psychologist, 44,* 513–524.

Hobfoll, S. E., Jackson, A. P., Lavin, J., Britton, P. J., & Shepherd, J. B. (1993). Safer sex knowledge, behavior, and attitudes of inner-city women. *Health Psychology, 12,* 481–488.

Hobfoll, S. E., Jackson, A. P., Lavin, J., Britton, P. J., & Shepherd, J. B. (1994). Reducing inner-city women's AIDS risk activities: A study of single, pregnant women. *Health Psychology, 13,* 397–403.

Hoff, C. C., Kegeles, S., Acree, M., Stall, R., Paul, J., Ekstrand, M., & Coates, T. (1997). Looking for men in all the wrong places...: HIV prevention small group programs do not reach high risk gay men. *AIDS, 11,* 829–831.

Holtgrave, D. R., & Kelly, J. A. (1996). Preventing HIV/AIDS among high-risk urban women: The cost-effectiveness of a behavioral group intervention. *American Journal of Public Health, 86,* 1442–1445.

Holtgrave, D. R., & Kelly, J. A. (1997). The cost-effectiveness of an HIV prevention intervention for gay men. *AIDS & Behavior, 1,* 173–180.

Holtgrave, D. R., Qualls, N., Curran, J., Valdiserri, R., Guinan, M., & Parra, W. (1995). An overview of the effectiveness an efficiency of HIV prevention programs. *Public Health Reports, 110,* 134–146.

Holtgrave, D. R., Valdiserri, R., Gerber, A. R., & Hinman, A. R. (1993). Human immunodeficiency virus counseling, testing, referral, and partner notification services: A cost-benefit analysis. *Archives of Internal Medicine, 153,* 1225–1230.

Holtgrave, D. R., Valdiserri, R., & West, G. (1994). Quantitative economic evaluations of HIV-related prevention and treatment services: A review. *Risk, Health, Safety, and Environment, 5,* 29–47.

Hospers, H., & Kok, G. (1995). Determinants of safe and risk-taking sexual behavior among gay men: A review. *AIDS Education and Prevention, 7,* 74–96.

Howard, D. (1997). 'Morning after:' HIV prevention outweighs psycho-babble. *Southern Voice,* p. 10.

Howland, J., Baker, D., Johnson, J., & Scaramucci, J. (1988). Teaching about AIDS in public school: Characteristics of early adopter communities in Massachusetts. *New York State Journal of Medicine, 88,* 62–65.

Ickovics, J. R., Morril, A. C., Beren, S. E., Walsh, U., & Rodin, J. (1994). Limited effects of HIV counseling and testing for women: A prospective study of behavioral and psychological consequences. *JAMA, 272,* 443–448.

Inciardi, J. A. (1994). HIV/AIDS risks among male, heterosexual noninjecting drug users who exchange crack for sex. In R. Battjes, Z. Sloboda, & W. Grace (Eds.), *The context of HIV risk among drug users and their sexual partners* (pp, 26–40). Washington, DC: NIDA.

Institute of Medicine. (1995). *Preventing HIV transmission: The role of sterile needles and bleach.* Washington, DC: National Academy Press.

International Working Group on Vaginal Microbicides. (1996). Recommendations for the development of vaginal microbicides. *AIDS, 10,* 1–6.

James, N. J., Bignell, C. J., & Gillies, P. A. (1991). The reliability of self-reported sexual behaviour. *AIDS, 5,* 333–336.

Janis, I. L., & Mann, L. (1977). *Decision making: A psychological analysis of conflict, choice, and commitment.* New York: The Free Press.

Jemmott, J. B., Jemmott, L. S., & Fong, G. T. (1992). Reductions in HIV risk-associated sexual behaviors among Black male adolescents: Effects of an AIDS prevention intervention. *American Journal of Public Health, 82,* 372–377.

Jemmott, L. S., Jemmott, J. B., & McCaffree, K. A. (1994). *Be proud! Be responsible: Strategies to empower youth to reduce their risk for AIDS.* New York: Select Media.

Johnson, E. H., Hinkle, Y., Gilbert, D., & Gant, L. M. (1992). Black males who always use condoms: Their attitudes, knowledge about AIDS, and sexual behavior. *Journal of the National Medical Association, 84,* 341–352.

Jones, J. L., Wykoff, R., Hollis, S., Longshore, S. T., Gamble, W., & Gunn, R. (1990). Partner acceptance of health department notification of HIV exposure, South Carolina. *JAMA, 264,* 1284–1285.

Jorgensen, S. R., Potts, V., & Camp, B. (1983). Project taking charge: Six-month follow-up of a pregnancy prevention program for early adolescents. *Family Relations, 42,* 401–406.

Joseph, J. G., Adib, M., Koopman, J. S., & Ostrow, D. G. (1990). Behavioral change in longitudinal studies: Adoption of condom use by homosexual/bisexual men. *American Journal of Public Health, 80,* 1513–1514.

Joseph, J. G., Montgomery, S., Emmons, C., Kirscht, J., Kessler, R., Ostrow, D., Wortman, C., O'Brien, K., Eller, M., & Eshleman, S. (1987). Perceived risk of AIDS: Assessing the behavioral and psychosocial consequences in a cohort of gay men. *Journal of Applied Social Psychology, 17,* 231–250.

Kalichman, S. C. (1994). Magic Johnson and public attitudes towards AIDS: A review of empirical findings. *AIDS Education and Prevention, 6,* 542–557.

Kalichman, S. C. (1995). *Understanding AIDS: A Guide for Mental Health Professionals.* Washington, DC: American Psychological Association.

Kalichman, S. C. (1996). HIV–AIDS education and prevention videotapes: Review of empirical findings and future directions. *Journal of Primary Prevention, 17,* 259–279.

Kalichman, S. C. (1997). *Post-exposure prophylaxis for HIV infection in gay and bisexual men: Implications for the future of HIV prevention.* Manuscript submitted for publication.

Kalichman, S. C. (1998). *Disclosure of HIV status and sexual practices of HIV seropositive men and women.* Manuscript submitted for publication.

Kalichman, S. C., Adair, V., Rompa, D., Multhauf, K., Johnson, J., & Kelly, J. (1994). Sexual sensation-seeking: Scale development and predicting AIDS-risk behavior among homosexually active men. *Journal of Personality Assessment, 62,* 385–397.

Kalichman, S. C., & Belcher, L. (1997). What the public is asking about AIDS: Conceptual and content analysis of questions asked of AIDS-information hotlines. *Health Education Research: Theory and Practice, 12,* 279–288.

Kalichman, S. C., Belcher, L., Cherry, C., & Williams, E. (1997). Primary prevention of sexually transmitted HIV infections: Transferring behavioral research to community programs. *Journal of Primary Prevention, 18,* 149–172.

Kalichman, S. C., Belcher, L., Cherry, C., Williams, E., & Allers, C. (1997). Human immunodeficiency virus (HIV) positive homeless men: Behavioral and social characteristics. *Journal of Social Distress and Homelessness, 6,* 303–318.

Kalichman, S. C., Belcher, L., Cherry, C., Williams, E. A., Sanders, M., & Allers, C. (in press). Risk for human immunodeficiency virus (HIV) infection and use of cocaine among indigent African-American men. *American Journal of Health Behavior.*

Kalichman, S. C., Carey, M. P., & Carey, K. B. (1996). Human immunodeficiency virus (HIV) risk among the seriously mentally ill. *Clinical Psychology: Science and Practice, 3,* 130–143.

Kalichman, S. C., Carey, M. P., & Johnson, B. T. (1996). Prevention of sexually transmitted HIV infection: Meta-analytic review and critique of the theory-based intervention outcome literature. *Annals of Behavioral Medicine, 18,* 6–15.

Kalichman, S. C., & Cherry, C. (1997). A skills-based *HIV-prevention intervention for African-American men.* United States Conferences on AIDS, Miami.

Kalichman, S. C., Cherry, C., Williams, E., Abush–Kirsh, T., Nachimson, D., Schaper, P., Belcher, L., & Smith, S. (1997). Oral sex anxiety, oral sexual behavior, and human immunodeficiency virus (HIV) risk perceptions among gay and bisexual men. *Journal of the Gay and Lesbian Medical Association, 1,* 161–168.

Kalichman, S. C., & Coley, B. (1995). Context framing to enhance HIV antibody testing messages targeted to African-American women. *Health Psychology, 14,* 247–254.

Kalichman, S. C., Greenberg, J., & Abel, G. G. (1997). Sexual compulsivity among HIV positive men who engage in high-risk sexual behavior with multiple partners: An exploratory study. *AIDS Care, 9,* 443–452.

Kalichman, S. C., Heckman, T., & Kelly, J. A. (1996). Sensation seeking, substance use, and HIV–AIDS risk behavior: Directional relationships among gay men. *Archives of Sexual Behavior, 25,* 141–154.

Kalichman, S. C., & Hospers, H. (1997). Efficacy of behavioral skills enhancement HIV risk reduction interventions in community settings. *AIDS, 11,* 191–199.

Kalichman, S. C., & Hunter, T. (1992). Disclosure of celebrity HIV infection: Effects on public attitudes. *American Journal of Public Health, 82,* 1374–1376.

Kalichman, S. C., Hunter, T. L., & Kelly, J. A. (1992). Perceptions of AIDS risk susceptibility among minority and nonminority women at risk for HIV infection. *Journal of Consulting and Clinical Psychology, 60,* 725–732.

Kalichman, S. C., Kelly, J. A., Hunter, T. L., Murphy, D. A., & Tyler, R. (1993). Culturally tailored HIV–AIDS risk-reduction messages targeted to African-American urban women: Impact on risk sensitization and risk reduction. *Journal of Consulting and Clinical Psychology, 61,* 291–295.

Kalichman, S. C., Kelly, J. A., Morgan, M., & Rompa, D. (1997). Fatalism, future outlook, current life satisfaction, and risk for human immunodeficiency virus (HIV) infection among gay and bisexual men. *Journal of Consulting and Clinical Psychology, 65,* 542–546.

Kalichman, S. C., Kelly, J. A., & Rompa, D. (1997). Continued high-risk sex among HIV seropositive men. *Health Psychology, 16,* 369–373.

Kalichman, S. C., Kelly, J. A., & Stevenson, L.Y. (1997). Priming effects of HIV risk assessments on related perceptions and behaviors: An experimental field study. *AIDS & Behavior, 1*, 3–8.

Kalichman, S. C., Roffman, R., Picciano, J., & Bolan, M. (1997). Sexual relationships and sexual risk behaviors among human immunodeficiency virus (HIV) seropositive gay and bisexual men seeking risk reduction services. *Professional Psychology: Research and Practice, 28*, 355–360.

Kalichman, S. C., Roffman, R., Picciano, J., & Bolan, M. (1997). *Risk for human immunodeficiency virus (HIV) infection among gay and bisexual men seeking HIV-prevention services and risks posed to their female partners.* Manuscript submitted for publication.

Kalichman, S. C., & Rompa, D. (1995). Sexually coerced and noncoerced gay and bisexual men: Factors relevant to risk for human immunodeficiency virus (HIV) infection. *Journal of Sex Research, 32*, 45–50.

Kalichman, S. C., Rompa, D., & Coley, B. (1996). Experimental component analysis of a behavioral HIV–AIDS prevention intervention for inner-city women. *Journal of Consulting and Clinical Psychology, 64*, 687–693.

Kalichman, S. C., Rompa, D., & Coley, B. (1997). Lack of positive outcomes from a cognitive-behavioral HIV–AIDS prevention intervention for inner-city men: Lessons from a controlled pilot study. *AIDS Education and Prevention, 9*, 299–313.

Kalichman, S. C., Rompa, D., & Muhammad, A. (1996). Psychological predictors of risk for human immunodeficiency virus (HIV) infection among low-income inner-city men: A community-based survey. *Psychology and Health, 12*, 493–503.

Kalichman, S. C., Russell, R. L., Hunter, T. L., & Sarwer, D. (1993). Earvin "Magic" Johnson's HIV-serostatus disclosure: Effects on men's perceptions of AIDS. *Journal of Consulting and Clinical Psychology, 61*, 887–891.

Kalichman, S. C., Schaper, P., Belcher, L., Abush–Kirsh, T., & Cherry, C. (1997). "It's like a regular part of gay life": Repeat HIV antibody testing among gay and bisexual men. *AIDS Education and Prevention, 9* (Suppl. B), 41–51.

Kalichman, S. C., Sikkema, K. J., Kelly, J. A., & Bulto, M. (1995). Use of a brief behavioral skills intervention to prevent HIV infection among chronic mentally ill adults. *Psychiatric Services, 46*, 275–280.

Kalichman, S. C., Somlai, A., Adair, V., & Weir, S. (1996). Psychological and social factors associated with HIV testing among sexually transmitted disease clinic patients: An exploratory study. *Psychology and Health, 11*, 593–604.

Kalichman, S. C., & Stevenson, L. Y. (1997). Risk factors for human immunodeficiency virus (HIV) infection among African-American women: A community-based survey. *Journal of Women's Health, 6*, 209–217.

Kamb, M., Douglas, J. M., Rhodes, F., Bolan, G., Iatesta, M., Peterman, T., Graziano, S., Killean, W., & Fishbein, M. (July, 1996). *A multi-center randomized controlled trial evaluating HIV prevention counseling (Project Respect): Preliminary results.* XI International Conference on AIDS, Vancouver.

Kane, S. (1991). HIV, heroin and heterosexual relations. *Social Science Medicine, 9*, 1037–1050.

Katchadourian, H. A. (1987). *Biological aspects of human sexuality* (3rd ed.). New York: Holt, Rinehart, & Winston.

Katz, M., & Gerberding, J. L. (1997). Post exposure treatment of people exposed to the human immunodeficiency virus through sexual contact or injection drug use. *New England Journal of Medicine, 336*, 1097–1100.

Katzenstein, D. A., Hammer, S. H., Hughes, M. D., Gundacker, H., Jackson, J. B., Fiscus, S., Rasheed, S., Elbeik, T., Reichman, R., Japour, A., Merigan, T. C., & Hirsch, M. S. (1996). The relation of virologic and immunologic to clinical outcomes after nucleoside therapy in HIV-infected adults with 200–500 CD4 cells per cubic millimeter. *The New England Journal of Medicine, 335*, 1091–1098.

Kauth, M. R., St. Lawrence, J. S., & Kelly, J. A. (1991). Reliability of retrospective assessments of sexual HIV risk behavior: A comparison of biweekly, 3-month, and 12-month self reports. *AIDS Education and Prevention, 3*, 207–214.

Kazdin, A. (1992). *Methodological issues and strategies in clinical research.* Washington, DC: American Psychological Association.

Keet, I. P. M., van Lent, N. A., Sandfort, T. G. M., Coutinho, R. A., & van Griensven, J. P. (1992). Orogenital sex and transmission of HIV among homosexual men. *AIDS, 6,* 223–226.

Kegeles, S. M., Hays, R. B., & Coates, T. J. (1996). The Mpowerment Project: A community-level HIV prevention intervention for young gay men. *American Journal of Public Health, 86,* 1129–1136.

Kelly, J. A. (1991). Changing the behavior of an HIV-seropositive man who practices unsafe sex. *Hospital and Community Psychiatry, 42,* 239–240, 264

Kelly, J. A., Heckman, T. G., & Helfrich, S. E. (1995). HIV risk factors and behaviors in a Milwaukee homeless shelter. *American Journal of Public Health, 85,* 1585.

Kelly, J. A., & Kalichman, S. C. (1995). Increased attention to human sexuality can improve HIV/AIDS prevention efforts: Key research issues and directions. *Journal of Consulting and Clinical Psychology, 63,* 907–918.

Kelly, J. A., Kalichman, S. C., & Rompa, D. (July, 1996). *Outcomes of a Randomized trial to promote consistent HIV risk reduction behavior change maintenance in an ethnically-diverse cohort of gay and bisexual men.* XI International Conference on AIDS, Vancouver.

Kelly, J. A., McAuliffe, T., Sikkema, K., Murphy, D., Somlai, A., Mulry, G., Miller, J., Stevenson, L., & Fernandez, I. (1997). Reduction in risk behavior among adults with severe mental illness who learned to advocate for HIV prevention. *Psychiatric Services, 48,* 1283–1288.

Kelly, J. A., Murphy, D. A., Bahr, G. R., Koob, J., Morgan, M., Kalichman, S. C., Stevenson, L.Y., Brasfield, T. L., Bernstein, B., & St. Lawrence, J. (1993). Factors associated with severity of depression among persons diagnosed with human immunodeficiency virus (HIV) infection. *Health Psychology, 12,* 215–219.

Kelly, J. A., Murphy, D. A., Roffman, R., Solomon, L., Winett, R., Stevenson, L., Koob, J., Ayotte, D., Flynn, B., Desiderato, L., Hauth, A., Lemke, A., Lombard, D., Morgan, M., Norman, A., Sikkema, K., Steiner, S., & Yaffe, D. (1992). Acquired immunodeficiency syndrome/human immunodeficiency virus risk behavior among gay men in small cities: Findings of a 16-city national sample. *Archives of Internal Medicine, 152,* 2293–2297.

Kelly, J. A., Murphy, D. A., Sikkema, K., McAuliffe, T., Roffman, R., Solomon, L., Winett, R., & Kalichman, S. C. (July, 1996). *Outcomes of a randomized controlled community-level HIV prevention intervention: Effects on behavior among at-risk gay men in 16 small US cities.* XI International Conference on AIDS, Vancouver.

Kelly, J. A., Murphy, D., Sikkema, K., McAuliffe, T., Roffman, R., Solomon, L., Winett, R., & Kalichman, S. C. (1997). Outcomes of a randomized controlled community-level HIV prevention intervention: effects on behavior among at-risk gay men in small U.S. cities. *Lancet, 350,* 1500–1505.

Kelly, J. A., Murphy, D. A., Washington, C. D., Wilson, T. S., Koob, J. J., Davis, D. R., Ledezma, G., & Davantes, B. (1994). The effects of HIV/AIDS intervention groups for high-risk women in urban clinics. *American Journal of Public Health, 84,* 1918–1922.

Kelly, J. A., & St. Lawrence, J. S. (1990). Behavioral group intervention to teach AIDS risk reduction skills. Treatment manual available from University of Mississippi Medical Center, Jackson, MS 39216.

Kelly, J. A., St. Lawrence, J. S., & Brasfield, T. L. (1991). Predictors of vulnerability to AIDS risk behavior relapse. *Journal of Consulting and Clinical Psychology, 59,* 163–166.

Kelly, J. A., St. Lawrence, J. S., Hood, H.V., & Brasfield, T. L. (1989). Behavioral intervention to reduce AIDS risk activities. *Journal of Consulting and Clinical Psychology, 57,* 60–67.

Kelly, J. A., & Stevenson, L. Y. (1995). *Opinion Leader HIV Prevention Training Manual.* Milwaukee, WI: Center for AIDS Intervention Research (CAIR) Medical College of Wisconsin.

Kennedy, C. A., Skurnick, J., Wan, J. Y., Quattrone, G., Sheffet, A., Quinones, M., Wang, W., & Louria, D. B. (1993). Psychological distress, drug and alcohol use in HIV-serodiscordant heterosexual couples. *AIDS, 7,* 1493–1499.

Kennedy, M., Scarlett, M., Duerr, A., & Chu, S. (1995). Assessing HIV risk among women who have sex with women: Scientific and communication issues. *Journal of the Medical Women's Association, 50,* 103–107.

Kingsley, L. A., Detels, R., Kaslow, R., Polk, B. F., Rinaldo, C. R., & Chmiel, J. (1987). Risk factors for seroconversion to human immunodeficiency virus among male homosexuals. *Lancet, 1,* 345–349.

Kippax, S., Crawford, J., Davis, M., Rodden, P., & Dowsett, G. (1993). Sustaining safe sex: A longitudinal sample of homosexual men. *AIDS, 7,* 257–263.

Kippax, S., Noble, J., Prestage, G., Crawford, J. M., Cambell, D., Baxter, D., and Cooper, D. (1997). Sexual negotiation in the AIDS era: Negotiated safety revisited. *AIDS, 11,* 191–197.

Kirby, D. (1995). A review of educational programs designed to reduce sexual risk-taking behaviors among school-aged youth in the United States. In Office of Technology Assessment, *The Effectiveness of AIDS Prevention Efforts* (pp. 158–235). Washington: American Psychological Association Office on AIDS.

Kirby, D., Short, L., Collins, J., Rugg, D., Kolbe, L., Howard, M., Miller, B., Sonenstein, F., & Zabin, L. S. (1994). School-based programs to reduce sexual risk behaviors: A review of effectiveness. *Public Health Reports, 109,* 339–360.

Koss, M. P., Gidycz, C. A., & Wisniewski, N. (1987). The scope of rape: Incidence and prevalence of sexual aggression and victimization in a national sample of higher education students. *Journal of Consulting and Clinical Psychology, 55,* 162–170.

Kotarba, J. A. (1990). Ethnography and AIDS: Returning to the streets. *Journal of Contemporary Ethnography, 19,* 259–270.

Kotler, P., & Roberto, E. (1989). *Social marketing: Strategies for changing public behavior.* New York: The Free Press.

Krupnick, J. L., Sotsky, S., Simmens, S., Moyer, J., Elkin, I., Watkins, J., & Pilkonis, P. (1996). The role of therapeutic alliance in psychotherapy and pharmocotherapy outcome: Findings from the National Institute of Mental Health treatment of depression collaborative research program. *Journal of Consulting and Clinical Psychology, 64,* 532–539.

Kuritzkes, D. R. (1996). Clinical significance of drug resistance in HIV-1 infection. *AIDS, 10* (Suppl. 5), S27–S31.

Landis, S. E., Schoenbach, V. J., Weber, D. J., Mittal, M., Krishan, B., Lewis, K., & Koch, G. G. (1992). Results of a randomized trial of partner notification in cases of HIV infection in North Carolina. *The New England Journal of Medicine, 326,* 101–106.

Latif, A. S., Katzenstein, D. A., Bassett, M. T., Houston, S., Emmanuel, J. C., & Marowa, E. (1989). Genital ulcers and transmission of HIV among couples in Zimbabwe. *AIDS, 3,* 519–523.

Laumann, E., Masi, C., & Zuckerman, E. (1997). Circumcision in the United States: Prevalence, prophylactic effects, and sexual practice. *JAMA, 277,* 1052–1057.

Lebow, J. M., O'Connell, J. J., Oddleifson, S., Gallagher, K. M., Seage, G. R., & Freedberg, K. A. (1995). AIDS among the homeless of Boston: A cohort study. *Journal of Acquired Immune Deficiency Syndromes and Human Retroviruses,* 292–296.

Leigh, B. C., & Stall, R. (1993). Substance use and risky sexual behavior for exposure to HIV: Issues in methodology, interpretation, and prevention. *American Psychologist, 48,* 1035–1045.

Lemp, G. F., Hirozawa, A. M., Givertz, D., Nieri, G. N., Anderson, L., Lindegren, M. L., Janssen, R. S., & Katz, M. (1994). Seroprevalence of HIV and risk behaviors among young homosexual and bisexual men. *Journal of the American Medical Association, 272,* 449–454.

Lemp, G. F., Payne, S. F., Neal, D., Temelso, T., & Rutherford, G. W. (1990). Survival trends for patients with AIDS. *JAMA, 263,* 402–406.

Leviton, L. C., & Schuh, R. G. (1991). Evaluation of outreach as a project element. *Evaluation Review, 15,* 420–440.

Levy, J. A. (1992). Viral and immunologic factors in HIV infection. In M. A. Sande & P. A. Volberding (Eds.), *The medical management of AIDS* (3rd ed.), (pp.18–32). Philadelphia: Saunders.

Lichtenstein, E., Glasgow, R. E., Lando, H. A., Ossip–Klein, D. J., & Boles, S. M. (1996). Telephone counseling for smoking cessation: Rationales and meta-analytic review of evidence. *Health Education Research: Theory & Practice, 11*, 243–257.

Lifson, A. R., O'Malley, P., Hessol, N. A., Buchbinder, S. P., Cannon, L., & Rutherford, G. (1990). HIV seroconversion in two homosexual men after receptive oral intercourse with ejaculation: Implications for counseling concerning safe sex. *American Journal of Public Health, 81*, 1509–1511.

Ling, J. C., Franklin, B., Lindsteadt, J., & Gearon, S. (1992). Social marketing: Its place in public health. In G. S. Omenn, J. E. Fielding, & L. B. Lave (Eds.), *Annual Review of Public Health, 13*, (pp. 341–362). Palo Alto, CA: Annual Review.

Lipsky, J. J. (1996). Antiretroviral drugs for AIDS. *Lancet, 348*, 800–803.

Lyman, D., Winkelstein, W., Ascher, M., & Levy, J. A. (1986). Minimal risk of transmission of AIDS-associated retrovirus infection by oral-genital contact. *JAMA, 255*, 1703.

Magura, S., Grossman, J. I., Lipton, D. S., Siddiqi, Q., Shapiro, J., Marion, I., & Amann, K. R. (1989). Determinants of needle sharing among intravenous drug users. *American Journal of Public Health, 79*, 459–462.

Maibach, E. W., Kreps, G. L., & Bonaguro, E. W. (1993). Developing strategic communication campaigns for HIV/AIDS prevention. In S. C. Ratzan (Ed.), *AIDS: Effective health communication for the 90s* (pp. 15–35). Washington, DC: Taylor & Francis.

Main, D. S., Iverson, D. C., McGloin, J., Banspach, S. W., Collins, K., Rugg, D., & Kolbe, L. J. (1994). Preventing HIV infection among adolescents: Evaluation of a school-based education program. *Preventing Medicine, 23*, 409–417.

Malow, R., West, J., Corrigan, S., Pena, J., & Cunningham, S. (1994). Outcome of psychoeducation for HIV risk reduction. *AIDS Education and Prevention, 6*, 113–125.

Mann, J., & Tarantola, D. (1996). *AIDS in the World II*. New York: Oxford Press.

Mantell, J. E., DiVittis, A. T., & Auerbach, M. I. (1997). *Evaluating HIV prevention interventions*. New York: Plenum.

Markowitz, M., Saag, M., Powderly, W. G., Hurley, A. M., Hsu, A., Valdes, J. M., Henry, D., Sattler, F., Marca, A. L., Leonard, J. M., & Ho, D. D. (1995). A preliminary study of ritonavir, an inhibitor of HIV-1 protease, to treat HIV-1 infection. *The New England Journal of Medicine, 333*, 1534–1539.

Marks, G., Richardson, J., Ruiz, M., & Maldonado, N. (1992). HIV-infected men's practices in notifying past sexual partners of infection risk. *Public Health Reports, 107*, 100–105.

Marks, G., Richardson, J. L., & Maldonado, N. (1991). Self-disclosure of HIV infection to sexual partners. *American Journal of Public Health, 81*, 1321–1323.

Marks, G., Ruiz, M. S., Richardson, J. L., Reed, D., Mason, H. R. C., Sotelo, M., & Turner, P. A. (1994). Anal intercourse and disclosure of HIV infection among seropositive gay and bisexual men. *Journal of Acquired Immune Deficiency Syndromes, 7*, 866–869.

Martin, D. J. (1992). Inappropriate lubricant use with condoms by homosexual men. *Public Health Reports, 107*, 468–473.

Mason, H., Marks, G., Simoni, J., Ruiz, M., & Richardson, J. (1995). Culturally sanctioned secrets? Latino men's nondisclosure of HIV infection to family, friends, and lovers. *Health Psychology, 14*, 6–12.

McCoy, C. B., Rivers, J. E., & Khoury, E. (1993). An emerging public health model for reducing AIDS related risk behavior among injection drug users and their sexual partners. *Drugs & Society, 7*, 143–159.

McCusker, J., Stoddard, A., & Hindin, R. (1996). Changes in HIV risk behavior following alternative residential programs for drug abuse treatment and AIDS education. *Annals of Epidemiology, 6*, 119–125.

McCusker, J., Stoddard, A. M., Mayer, K. H., Zapka, J., Morrison, C., & Saltzman, S. P. (1988). Effects of HIV antibody test knowledge on subsequent sexual behaviors in a

Normand, J., Vlahov, D., & Moses, L. (1995). *Preventing HIV transmission: The role of sterile needles and bleach.* Washington, DC: National Academy Press.

Nyamathi, A. M., Bennett, C., & Leake, B. (1995). Predictors of maintained high-risk behaviors among impoverished women. *Public Health Reports, 110,* 600–606.

Nyamathi, A. M., Flaskerud, J., Bennett, C., Leake, B., & Lewis, C. (1994). Evaluation of two AIDS education programs for impoverished Latina women. *AIDS Education and Prevention, 6,* 296–309.

O'Brien, T., Busch, M., Donegan, E., Ward, J., Wong, L., Samson, S., Perkins, H., Altman, R., Stoneburner, R., & Holmberg, S. (1994). Heterosexual transmission of human immunodeficiency virus type 1 from transfusion recipients to their sex partners. *Journal of Acquired Immune Deficiency Syndromes, 7,* 705–710.

O'Donnell, L., Doval, A. S., Duran, R., & O'Donnell, C. R. (1995). Predictors of condom acquisition after an STD clinic visit. *Family Planning Perspectives, 27,* 29–33.

Office of Technology Assessment. (1995). *The Effectiveness of AIDS Prevention Efforts.* Washington: American Psychological Association Office on AIDS.

O'Hara, P., Messick, B. J., Fitchner, R. R., & Parris, D. (1996). A peer-led AIDS prevention program for students in an alternative school. *Journal of School Health, 66,* 176–182.

Ostrow, D., DiFranceisco, W., Chmeil, J., Wagstaff, D., & Wesch J. (1995). A case-control study of human immunodeficiency virus type-1 seroconversion and risk-related behaviors in the Chicago MACS/CCS cohort, 1984–1992. *American Journal of Epidemiology, 142,* 1–10.

Ostrow, D., DiFrancheisco, W., & Kalichman, S. C. (1997). Sexual adventurism and high-risk sexual behavior among gay and bisexual men at risk for HIV infection. *AIDS & Behavior.*

Ostrow, D. G., Beltran, E. D., Joseph, J. G., DiFranceisco, W., Wesch, J., & Chmiel, J. (1993). Recreational drugs and sexual behavior in the Chicago MACS/CCS cohort of homosexually active men. *Journal of Substance Abuse, 5,* 311–325.

Ostrow, D. G., & Kessler, R.C. (1993). *Methodological issues in AIDS behavioral research.* New York: Plenum.

Ostrow, D. G., Kessler, R. C., Stover, E., & Pequegnat, W. (1993). Design, measurement, and analysis issues in AIDS mental health research. In D. G. Ostrow & R. C. Kessler (Eds.), *Methodological issues in AIDS behavioral research* (pp. 1–16). New York: Plenum.

Owens, D. K., Nease, R. F., & Harris, R. A. (1996). Cost-effectiveness of HIV screening in acute care settings. *Archives of Internal Medicine, 156,* 394–404.

Padian, N., Marquis, L., Francis, D. P., Anderson, R. E., Rutherford, G., O'Malley, P. M., & Winkelstein, W. (1987).Male-to-female transmission of human immunodeficiency virus. *Journal of the American Medical Association, 258,* 788–790.

Padian, N. S. (1990). Sexual histories of heterosexual couples with one HIV-infected partner. *The American Journal of Public Health, 80,* 990–991.

Padian, N. S., O'Brien, T. R., Chang, Y. C., Glass, S., & Francis, D. P. (1993). Prevention of heterosexual transmission of human immunodeficiency virus through couple counseling. *Journal of Acquired Immune Deficiency Syndromes, 6,* 1043–1048.

Padian, N. S., Shiboski, S. C., & Jewell, N. P. (1991). Female-to-male transmission of human immunodeficiency virus. *Journal of the American Medical Association, 266,* 1664–1667.

Payne, J. G., & Mercuri, K. A. (1993). Crisis in communication: Coverage of Magic Johnson's AIDS disclosure. In S. C. Ratzan (Ed.), *AIDS: Effective health communication for the 90s* (pp. 151–172). Washington, DC: Taylor & Francis.

Pendergrast, R. A., DuRant, R. H., & Gaillard, G. L. (1992). Attitudinal and behavioral correlates of condom use in urban adolescent males. *Journal of Adolescent Health, 13,* 133–139.

Penner, L. A., & Fritzsche, B. A. (1993). Magic Johnson and reactions to people with AIDS: A natural experiment. *Journal of Applied Social Psychology, 23,* 1035–1050.

Perry, S. W., & Markowitz, J. C. (1988). Counseling for HIV testing. *Hospital and Community Psychiarty, 39,* 731–739.

Perry, S., Jacobsberg, L., Card, C. A., Ashman, T., Frances, A., & Fishman, B. (1993). Severity of psychiatric symptoms after HIV testing. *American Journal of Psychiatry, 150,* 775–779.

Persky, H., Strauss, D., Lief, H. I., Miller, W. R., & O'Brien, C. P. (1981). Effects of the research process on human sexual behavior. *Journal of Psychiatry Research, 16,* 41–52.

Petersen, L. R., Doll, L., White, C., Chu, S., & the HIV Blood Donor Study Group. (1992). No evidence for female-to-female HIV transmission among 960,000 female blood donors. *Journal of Acquired Immune Deficiency Syndromes, 5,* 853–855.

Peterson, J. L., Coates, T. J., Catania, J., Hauck, W. W., Acree, M., Daigle, D., Hillard, B., Middleton, L., & Hearst, N. (1996). Evaluation of an HIV risk reduction intervention among African-American homosexual and bisexual men. *AIDS, 10,* 319–325.

Phillips, K., Flatt, S., Morrison, K., & Coates, T. (1995). Potential use of home HIV testing. *New England Journal of Medicine, 332,* 1308–1310.

Phillips, K., Paul, J., Kegeles, S., Stall, R., Hoff, C., & Coates, T. (1995). Predictors of repeat HIV testing among gay and bisexual men. *AIDS, 9,* 769–775.

Pinkerton, S. D., Holtgrave, D. R., & Valdiserri, R. O. (1997). Cost-effectiveness of HIV prevention skills training for men who have sex with men. *AIDS, 11,* 347–357.

Polinko, P., Bradley, W. F., Molyneaux, B., & Lukoff, C. (1995). HIV in health care workers: Managing fear through a telephone information line. *Social Work, 40,* 819–822.

Prochaska, J. O., DiClemente, C. C., & Norcross, J. C. (1992). In search of how people change. *American Psychologists, 47,* 1102–1113.

Prochaska, J. O., Redding, C. A., Harlow, C. A., Rossi, J. S., & Velicer, W. F. (1994). The transtheoretical model of change and HIV prevention: A review. *Health Education Quarterly, 21,* 471–486.

Pulley, L. V., McAlister, A. L., Kay, L. S., & O'Reilly, K. (1996). Prevention campaigns for hard-to-reach populations at risk for HIV infection: Theory and implementation. *Health Education Quarterly, 23,* 488–496.

Quadland, M. C. (1985). Compulsive sexual behavior: Definition of a problem and an approach to treatment. *Journal of Sex and Marital Therapy, 11,* 121–132.

Quadland, M. C., & Shattls, W. D. (1987). AIDS, sexuality, and sexual control. *Journal of Homosexuality, 14,* 277–298.

Quinn, T. C., Glaser, D., Cannon, R. O., Matuszak, D. L., Dunning, R. W., & Kline, M. S. (1988). Human immunodeficiency virus infection among patients attending clinics for sexually transmitted diseases. *New England Journal of Medicine, 318,* 197–203.

Ratner, M. S. (1993). *Crack pipe as pimp: An ethnographic investigation of sex-for-crack exchanges.* New York: Lexington.

Reading, A. E. (1983). A comparison of the accuracy and reactivity of methods of monitoring male sexual behavior. *Journal of Behavioral Assessment, 5,* 11–23.

Reed, G. M., & Collins, B. E. (1994). Mental health research and service delivery: A three communities model. *Psychosocial Rehabilitation Journal, 17,* 69–74.

Remien, R. H., Carballo–Dieguez, A., & Wagner, G. (1995). Intimacy and sexual behavior in serodiscordant male couples. *AIDS Care, 7,* 429–438.

Rhodes, T. J., Donoghoe, M. C., Hunter, G. M., & Stimson, G. V. (1993). Continued risk behavior among HIV positive drug injectors in London: Implications for intervention. *Addiction, 88,* 1553–1560.

Richters, J., Donovan, B., & Gerofi, J. (1993). How often do condoms break or slip off in use? *Internation Journal of STD & AIDS, 4,* 90–94.

Richters, J., Gerofi, J., & Donovan, B. (1995). Why do condoms break or slip off in use? An exploratory study. *International Journal of STD & AIDS, 6,* 11–18.

Robins, A. G., Dew, M. A., Davidson, S., Penkower, L., Becker, J. T., & Kingsley, L. (1994). Psychosocial factors associated with risky sexual behavior among HIV-seropositive gay men, *AIDS Education and Prevention, 6,* 483–492.

Roffman, R. A., Picciano, J. F., Ryan, R., Beadnell, B., Fisher, D., Downey, L., & Kalichman, S. C. (1997). HIV prevention group counseling delivered by telephone: An efficacy trial with gay and bisexual men. *AIDS & Behavior, 1,* 137–154.

Roffman, R. A., Picciano, J., Wickizer, L., Bolan, M., & Ryan, R. (in press). Anonymous enrollment in AIDS prevention group counseling: Facilitating the participation of gay and bisexual men. *Journal of Social Service Research.*

Rogers, C. R. (1961). *On becoming a person.* Boston: Houghton Mifflin Company.

Rogers, E. M. (1995a). Diffusion of drug abuse prevention programs: Spontaneous diffusion, agenda setting, and reinvention. In T. E. Baker, S. L. David, & G. Soucy (Eds.), *Reviewing the behavioral science knowledge base on technology transfer* (pp. 90–100). Washington, DC: National Institute on Drug Abuse.

Rogers, E. M. (1995b). *Diffusion of Innovations,* (4th ed.). New York: The Free Press

Rojanapithayakorn, W., & Hanenberg, R. (1996). The 100% condom program in Thailand. *AIDS, 10,* 1–7.

Rosenberg, M. J., Holmes, K. K., & the World Health Organization Working Group on Virucides. (1993). Virucides in prevention of HIV infection: Research priorities. *Sexually Transmitted Diseases, 20,* 41–44.

Rosenberg, M. J., Waugh, M. S., Soloman, H. W., & Lyszkowski, A. D. L. (1996). The male polyurethane condom: A review of current knowledge. *Contraception, 53,* 141–146.

Rosenstock, M., Strecher, V., & Becker, M. (1994). The health belief model and HIV risk behavior change. In R. DiClemente & J. Peterson (Eds.), *Preventing AIDS: Theories, methods, and behavioral interventions* (pp. 5–24). New York: Plenum.

Ross, M. W. (1987). Problems associated with condom use in homosexual men. *American Journal of Public Health, 77,* 877.

Ross, M. W. (1988). Attitudes toward condoms as AIDS prophylaxis in homosexual men: Dimensions and measurement. *Psychology and Health, 2,* 291–299.

Ross, M. W. (1992). Attitudes toward condoms and condom use: A review. *International Journal of STD & AIDS, 3,* 10–16.

Rotello, G. (1997). *Sexual ecology.* New York: Dutton.

Rothenberg, K. H., & Paskey, S. (1995). The risk of domestic violence and women with HIV infection: Implications for partner notification, public policy, and the law. *American Journal of Public Health, 85,* 1569–1576.

Rotheram-Borus, M. J., Koopman, C., & Haignere, C. (1991). Reducing HIV sexual risk behaviors among runaway adolescents. *JAMA, 266,* 1237–1241.

Rotheram-Borus, M. J., Reid, H., & Rosario, M. (1994). Factors mediating changes in sexual HIV risk behaviors among gay and bisexual male adolescents. *American Journal of Public Health, 84,* 1938–1946.

Rothspan, S., & Read, S. J. (1996). Present versus future time perspective and HIV risk among heterosexual college students. *Health Psychology, 15,* 131–134.

Royce, R. A., Sena, A., Cates, W., & Cohen, M. (1997). Sexual transmission of HIV. *New England Journal of Medicine, 336,* 1072–1078.

Saag, M. S. (1992). AIDS testing: Now and in the future. In M. A. Sande & P. A. Volberding (Eds.), *The medical management of AIDS* (3rd 3d.), (pp. 33–53). Philadelphia: Saunders.

Sacco, W. P., Levine, B., Reed, D. L., & Thompson, K. (1991). Attitudes about condom use as an AIDS-relevant behavior: Their factor structure and relation to condom use. *Psychological Assessment, 3,* 265–272.

Samuel, M. C., Hessol, N., Shiboski, S., Eagel, R., Speed, T. P., & Winkelstein, W. (1993). Factors associated with human immunodeficiency virus seroconversion in homosexual men in three San Francisco cohort studies, 1984–1989. *Journal of AIDS, 6,* 303–312.

San Francisco AIDS Foundation. (1994). *AIDS hotline training manual.* San Francisco: author.

Santelli, J. S., Davis, M., Celentano, D. D., Crump, A. D., & Burwell, L. G. (1995). Combined use of condoms with other contraceptive methods among inner-city Baltimore women. *Family Planning Perspectives, 27,* 74–78.

Saracco, A., Musicco, M., Nicilosi, A., Angarano, G., Arici, C., Gavazzeni, G., Costigliola, P., Gafa, S., Gervasoni, C., Luzzati, R., Piccinino, F., Puppo, F., Salassa, B., Sinicco, A., Stellini, R., Tirelli, U., Turbessi, G., Vigevani, G., Visco, G., Zerboni, R., &

Lazzarin, A. (1993). Man-to-woman sexual transmission of HIV: Longitudinal study of 434 steady sexual partners of infected men. *Journal of Acquired Immune Deficiency Syndromes, 6*, 497–502.

Schaalma, H., Kok, G., & Paulusses, T. (1996). HIV behavioural interventions in young people in the Netherlands. *International Journal of STD & AIDS, 7*, 43–46.

Schacker, T., Collier, A., Hughes, J., Shea, T., & Corey, L. (1996). Clinical and epidemiological features of primary HIV infection. *Annals of Internal Medicine, 125*, 257–264.

Schechter, M. T., Boyko, W., Douglas, B., & The Vancouver Lymphadenopathy-AIDS study: 6 (1985). HIV seroconversion in a cohort of homosexual men. *Canadian Medical Association Journal, 135*, 1355–1360.

Schilling, R. F., El–Bassel, N., Hadden, B., & Gilbert, L. (1995). Skills-training groups to reduce HIV transmission and drug use among methadone patients. *Social Work, 40*, 91–101.

Schnell, D., Higgins, D., Wilson, R., Goldbaum, G., Cohn, D., & Wolitski, R. (1992). Men's disclosure of HIV test results to male primary sex partners. *American Journal of Public Health, 82*, 1675–1676.

Schnell, D. J., Galavotti, C., Fishbein, M., & Chan, D. K–S. (1996). Measuring the adoption of consistent use of condoms using the stages of change model. *Public Health Reports, 111*, (Suppl. 1), 59–68.

Schoenbaum, E. E., Weber, M. P., Vermund, S., & Gayle, H. (1990). HIV antibody in persons screened for syphilis: Prevalence in a New York City emergency room and primary care clinics. *Sexually Transmitted Diseases, 17*, 190–193.

Schofield, J., & Pavelchak, M. (1985). The day after: The impact of a media event. *American Psychologist, 40*, 542–548.

Schooley, R. (1992). Anti-retroviral chemotherapy. In G. P. Wormser (Ed.), *AIDS and other manifestations of HIV infection* (2nd ed.), (pp. 609–624). New York: Raven.

Schopper, D., & Vercauteren, G. (1996). Testing for HIV at home: What are the issues? *AIDS, 10*, 1455–1465.

Schoub, B. D. (1993). *AIDS & HIV in perspective*. New York: Cambridge University Press.

Schwarcz, S. K., Kellogg, T., Kohn, R., Katz, M., Lemp, G., & Bolan, G. (1995). Temporal trends in human immunodeficiency virus seroprevalence and sexual behavior at the San Francisco Municipal Sexually Transmitted Disease Clinic, 1989–1992. *American Journal of Epidemiology, 142*, 314–322.

Schwarz, R. M. (1994). *The skilled facilitator: Practical wisdom for developing effective groups*. San Francisco: Jossey-Bass.

Scott, S. A., & Vangsnes, N. (November, 1995). *Personal dilemmas/individual decisions educating 'anonymous' about HIV/AIDS.* Paper presented at the Convention of the American Public Health Association, San Diego.

Seage, G. R., Mayer, K. H., & Horsburgh, C. R., Jr. (1993). Risk of human immunodeficiency virus infection from unprotected receptive anal intercourse increases with decline in immunologic status of infected partners. *American Journal of Epidemiology, 137*, 899–908.

Seal, D. W., & Agostinelli, G. (1994). Individual differences associated with high-risk sexual behaviours: Implications for intervention programmes. *AIDS Care, 6*, 393–397.

Seed, J., Allen, S., Mertens, T., Hudes, E., Serufilira, A., Carael, M., Karita, E., van de Perre, P., & Nsengumuremyi, F. (1995). Male circumcision, sexually transmitted disease, and risk of HIV. *Journal of Acquired Immune Deficiency Syndromes, 8*, 83–90.

Shervington, D. O. (1993). The acceptability of the female condom among low-income African-American women. *The Journal of the National Medical Association, 85*, 341–347.

Sikkema, K. J., & Kelly, J. A. (1995). *Community Intervention to reduce AIDS risk behavior: A prevention program for women living in housing developments.* Milwaukee: Center for AIDS Intervention Research Department of Psychiatry and Behavioral Medicine.

Sibthorpe, B., Fleming, D., & Gould, J. (1994). Self-help groups: A key to HIV risk reduction for high-risk injection drug users? *Journal of Acquired Immune Deficiency Syndromes, 7,* 595–598.

Sikkema, K. J., Koob, J., Cargill, V., Kelly, J. A., Desiderato, L., & Roffman, R. (1995). Levels and predictors of HIV risk behavior among women living in low-income housing developments. *Public Health Reports, 6,* 707–713.

Sikkema, K. J., Winett, R. A., & Lombard, D. N. (1995). Development and evaluation of an HIV-risk reduction program for female college students. *AIDS Education and Prevention, 7*(2), 145–159.

Simon, P. A., Weber, M., Ford, W., Cheng, F. & Kerndt, P. (1996). Reasons for HIV antibody test refusal in a heterosexual sexually transmitted disease clinic populations. *AIDS, 10,* 1549–1553.

Simoni, J. M., Mason, H. R. C., Marks, G., Ruiz, M. S., Reed, D., & Richardson, J. L. (1995). Women's self-disclosure of HIV infection: Rates, reasons, & reactions. *Journal of Consulting and Clinical Psychology, 63,* 474–478.

Simpson, D. D., Camacho, L. M., Vogtsberger, K. N., Williams, M. L., Stephens, R. C., Jones, A., & Watson, D. D. (1994). Reducing AIDS risks through community outreach interventions for drug injectors. *Psychology of Addictive Behaviors, 8,* 86–101.

Singh, B. K., Koman, J. J., III., Catan, V. M., Souply, K. L., Birkel, R. C., & Goolaszewski, T. J. (1993). Sexual risk behavior among injection drug-using human immunodeficiency virus positive clients. *The International Journal of the Addictions, 28,* 735–747.

Siska, M., Jason, J., Murdoch, P., Yang, W. S., & Donovan, R. J. (1992). Recall of AIDS public service announcements and their impact on the ranking of AIDS as a national problem. *American Journal of Public Health, 82,* 1029–1032.

Smith, P. F., Mikl, J., Hyde, S., & Morse, D. L. (1991). The AIDS epidemic in New York State. *American Journal of Public Health, 81,* 54–60.

Sobo, E. J. (1993). Inner-city women and AIDS: The psycho-social benefits of Unsafe sex. *Culture, Medicine and Psychiatry, 17,* 455–485.

Soper, D. E., Shoupe, D., Shangold, G. A., Shangold, M. M., Gutmann, J., & Mercer, L. (1993). Prevention of Vaginal Trichomoniasis by compliant use of the female condom. *Sexually Transmitted Diseases, 20*(3), 137–139.

Soto–Ramirez, L., Renjifo, B., McLane, M., Marlink, R., O'Hara, C., Sutthent, R., Wasi, C., Vithayasai, P., Vithayasai, V., Apichartpiyakul, C., Auewarakul, P., Cruz, V., Chui, D., Osathanondh, R., Mayer, K., Lee, T., & Essex, M. (1996). HIV-1 langerhans cell tropism associated with heterosexual transmission of HIV. *Science, 271,* 1291–1293.

Southern Voice. (1996, April 4). *Oral sex has little HIV risk, gay doctors say.* Author, p.12.

Stall, R., McKusick, L., Wiley, J., Coates, T. J., & Ostrow, D. G. (1986). Alcohol and drug use during sexual activity and compliance with safe sex guidelines for AIDS. *Health Education Quarterly, 13,* 359–371.

Steiner, M., Trussell, J., Glover, L., Joanis, C., Spruyt, A., & Dorflinger, L. (1994). Standardized protocols for condom breakage and slippage trials: A proposal. *American Journal of Public Health, 84,* 1897–1900.

Steiner, S., Lemke, A., & Roffman, R. (1994). Risk behavior for HIV transmission among gay men surveyed in Seattle bars. *Public Health Reports, 109,* 563–566.

Sterk–Elifson, C. (1993). Outreach among drug users: Combining the role of ethnographic field assistant and health educator. *Human Organization, 52,* 162–168.

Stevenson, H. C., & Davis, G. (1994). Impact of culturally sensitive AIDS video education on the AIDS risk knowledge of African-American adolescents. *AIDS Education and Prevention, 6,* 40–52.

St. Lawrence, J. S., & Brasfield, T. (1995). HIV risk behavior among homeless adults. *AIDS Education and Prevention, 7,* 22–31.

St. Lawrence, J. S., Eldridge, G., Shelby, M., Little, C., Brasfield, T., & O'Bannon, R. (1997). HIV risk reduction for incarcerated women: A comparison of brief interventions based on two theoretical models. *Journal of Consulting and Clinical Psychology, 65,* 504–509.

St. Lawrence, J. S., Jefferson, K. W., Alleyne, E., & Brasfield, T. L. (1995). Comparison of education versus behavioral skills training interventions in lowering sexual HIV-risk behavior of substance-dependent adolescents. *Journal of Consulting and Clinical Psychology, 63,* 154–157.

St. Lawrence, J. S., Reitman, D., Jefferson, K., Alleyne, E., Brasfield, T., Shirley, A. (1994). Factor structure and validation of an adolescent version of the condom attitude scale: An instrument for measuring adolescents' attitudes toward condoms. *Psychological Assessment, 6,* 352–359.

Stokes, J. P., McKirnan, D. J., & Burzette, B. G. (1993). Sexual behavior, condom use, disclosure of sexuality, and stability of sexual orientation in bisexual men. *The Journal of Sex Research, 30,* 203–213.

STOP AIDS Project. (1995). *Facilitator training manual.* San Francisco: Author.

St. Pierre, T. L., Mark, M. M., Kaltreider, D. L., & Aikin, K. J. (1995). A 27-month evaluation of a sexual activity prevention program in Boys & Girls Clubs across the nation. *Family Relations, 44,* 69–77.

Susser, E., Valencia, E., Berkman, A., Sohler, N., Conover, S., Torrres, J., Betne, P., Felix, A., & Miller, S. (1996). *HIV risk reduction in impaired populations: A controlled trial among homeless men.* Unpublished manuscript, Columbia University, New York.

Susser, E., Valencia, E., & Miller, M. (1995). Sexual behavior of homeless mentally ill men at risk for HIV. *American Journal of Psychiatry, 152,* 583–587.

Susser, E., Valencia, E., & Torres, J. (1994). Sex, games, and videotapes: An HIV-prevention intervention for men who are homeless and mentally ill. *Psychosocial Rehabilitation Journal, 17*(4), 31–40.

Tanfer, K., Grady, W. R., Klepinger, D. H., & Billy, J. O. (1993). Condom use among US men, 1991. *Family Planning Perspectives, 25,* 61–66.

Taylor, D. D., & Henderson, K. (1992). AIDS and Ontario's public education campaign: A social marketing calamity. *Canadian Journal of Administrative Sciences, 9,* 58–65.

Temple, M. T., & Leigh, B. C. (1992). Alcohol consumption and unsafe sexual behavior in discrete events. *Journal of Sex Research, 29,* 207–219.

Temple, M. T., Leigh, B. C., & Schafer, J. (1993). Unsafe sexual behavior and alcohol use at the event level: Results of a national survey. *Journal of Acquired Immune Deficiency Syndromes, 6,* 393–401.

Tenkasi, R. V., & Mohrman, S. A. (1995). Technology transfer as a collaborative learning. In T. E. Backer, S. L. David, & G. Soucy (Eds.), *Reviewing the behavioral science knowledge base on technology transfer* (pp. 147–168). Rockville, MD: National Institute on Drug Abuse.

Thompson, J. P., Yager, T., & Martin, J. L. (1993). Estimated condom failure and frequency of condom use among gay men. *American Journal of Public Health, 83,* 1409–1413.

Tindall, B., Swanson, C., Donovan, B., & Cooper, D. (1989). Sexual practices and condom usage in a cohort of homosexual men in relation to human immunodeficiency virus status. *The Medical Journal of Australia, 151,* 318–322.

Torian, L.V., Weisfuse, I. B., Makki, H. A., Benson, D., DiCamillo, L., Patel, P., & Toribio, F. (1996). Trends in HIV seroprevalence in men who have sex with men: New York City Department of Health sexually transmitted disease clinics, 1988–1993. *AIDS, 10,* 187–192.

Trotter, R. T., Bowen, A. M., Baldwin, J. A., & Price, L. J. (1996). The efficacy of network-based HIV/AIDS risk reduction program in midsized towns in the United States. *Journal of Drug Issues, 26,* 591–605.

Trussell, J., Hatcher, R. A., Cates, W., Stewart, F. H., & Kost, K. (1990). Contraceptive failure in the United States: An update. *Studies of Family Planning, 21,* 51–54.

Trussell, J. F., Warner, D. L., & Hatcher R. A. (1992b). Condom slippage and breakage rates. *Family Planning Perspective, 24,* 20–23.

UNAIDS. (1997). Implications of HIV variability for transmission. Scientific and policy issues. *AIDS, 11,* UNAIDS1–UNAIDS15.

Upchurch, D. M., Ray, P., Reichart, C., Celentano, D. D., Quinn, T., & Hook, E. W. (1992). Prevalence and patterns of condom use among patients attending a sexually transmitted disease clinic. *Sexually Transmitted Diseases, 19*, 175–180.

Urassa, M., Todd, J., Boerma, T., Hayes, R. & Isingo, R. (1997). Male circumcision and susceptibility to HIV infection among men in Tanzania. *AIDS, 11*, 73–80.

Valdisseri, R. O., Arena, V. C., Proctor, D., & Bonati, F. A. (1989). The relationships between women's attitudes about condoms and their use: Implications for condom promotion programs. *American Journal of Public Health, 79*(4), 499–501.

Valdiserri, R. O., Aultman, T., & Curran, J. (1995). Community planning: A national strategy to improve HIV prevention programs. *Journal of Community Health, 20*, 87–100.

Valdiserri, R. O., Lyter, D., Leviton, L., Callahan, C. N., Kingsley, L. A., & Rinaldo, C. R. (1989). AIDS prevention in homosexual and bisexual men: Results of a randomized trial evaluating two risk reduction interventions. *AIDS, 3*, 21–26.

Valdiserri, R. O., Moore, M., Gerber, A. R., Campbell, C. H., Dillon, B. A., & West, G. R. (1993). A study of clients returning for counseling after HIV testing: Implications for improving rates of return. *Public Health Reports, 108*, 12–18.

Valentine, J., & Wright–DeAgüero, L. K. (1996). Defining the components of street outreach for HIV prevention: The contact and the encounter. *Public Health Reports, 111*, (Suppl. 1), 69–74.

Vermund, S. H. (1996). Limitations of characterization of heterosexual transmission risk: Commentary on the models of Downs and De Vincenzi. *Journal of Acquired Immune Deficiency Syndromes, 11*, 385–387.

Waldorf, D., & Lauderback, D. (1993). Condom failure among male sex workers in San Francisco. *AIDS & Public Policy Journal, 8*, 79–90.

Walter, H. J., & Vaughan, R. D. (1993). Aids risk reduction among a multiethnic sample of urban high school students. *Journal of the American Medical Association, 270*, 725–730.

Wandersman, A., Morrissey, E. Seybolt, D., Nation, M., Crusto, C., & Davino, K. (1997). *Toward a framework for bridging the gap between science and practice in prevention: A focus on evaluator and practitioner perspectives.* Unpublished manuscript, University of South Carolina.

Wass, H., Miller, D., & Thornton, G. (1990). AIDS education in the U. S. public schools. *AIDS Education and Prevention,2*, 213–219.

Waterman, C. K., Dawson, L. J., & Bologna, M. J. (1989). Sexual coercion in gay male and lesbian relationships: Predictors and implications for support services. *The Journal of Sex Research, 26*, 118–124.

Watters, J., & Biermacki, P. (1989). Targeted sampling: Options for the study of hidden populations. *Social Problems, 36*, 416–430.

Webb, G. R., Redman, S., Gibberd, R. W., & Sanson–Fisher, R. W. (1991). The reliability and stability of a quantity-frequency method and a diary method of measuring alcohol consumption. *Drug and Alcohol Dependence, 27*, 223–231.

Weeks, K., Levy, S. R., Zhu, C., Perhats, C., Handler, A., & Flay, B. R. (1995). Impact of a school-based AIDS prevention program on young adolescents' self-efficacy skills. *Health Education Research Theory and Practice, 10*, 329–344.

Weinstein, B. (1997). Public health department perspective. *AIDS and Behavior, 1*, 205–206.

Weir, S., Feldblum, P., Roddy, & Zekeng, L. (1994). Gonorrhea as a risk factor for HIV acquisition. *AIDS, 8*, 165–168.

Wellman, M. C. (1993). An AIDS hotline: Analysis of callers, presenting problems, and social factors. *Journal of Applied Social Psychology, 23*, 1111–1123.

Wells, E. A., Calsyn, D. A., & Saxon, A. J. (1993). Using drugs to facilitate sexual behavior is associated with sexual variety among injection drug users. *Journal of Nervous and Mental Diseases, 181*, 626–631.

Wenger, N. S., Greenberg, J. M., Hilborne, L. H., Kusseling, F., Mangotich, M., & Shapiro, M. F. (1992). Effect of HIV antibody testing and AIDS education on communication about HIV risk and sexual behavior. *Annals of Internal Medicine, 117*, 905–911.

Wenger, N. S., Kusseling, F. S., Beck, K., & Shapiro, M. F. (1994). Sexual behavior of individuals infected with the human immunodeficiency virus: The need for intervention. *Archives of Internal Medicine, 154*, 1849–1854.

Wenger, N. S., Linn, L., Epstein, M., & Shapiro, M. (1991). Reduction of high-risk sexual behavior among heterosexuals undergoing HIV antibody testing: A randomized clinical trial. *American Journal of Public Health, 81*, 1580–1585.

West, S. G., Aiken, L. S., & Todd, M. (1993). Probing the effects of individual components in multiple component prevention programs. *American Journal of Community Psychology, 21*, 571–605.

Wiebel, W. (1993). *The indigenous leader outreach model: Intervention manual.* Rockville, MD: National Institute on Drug Abuse.

Williams, M. L. (1990). HIV seroprevalence among male IVDUs in Houston, Texas. *American Journal of Public Health, 80*, 1507–1508.

Wilson, T. E., Jaccard, J., Levinson, R., Minkoff, H., & Endias, R. (1996). Testing for HIV and other sexually transmitted diseases: Implications for risk behavior in women. *Health Psychology, 15*, 252–260.

Winett, R. A., Altman, D. G., & King, A. C. (1990). Conceptual and strategic foundations for effective media campaigns for preventing the spread of HIV infection. *Evaluation and Program Planning, 13*, 91–104.

Winett, R. A., Anderson, E., Desiderato, L., Solomon, L., Perry, M., Kelly, J., Sikkema, K., Roffman, R., Norman, A., Lombard, D., & Lombard, T. (1995). Enhancing social diffusion theory as a basis for prevention intervention: A conceptual and strategic framework. *Applied and Preventive Psychology, 4*, 233–245.

Wingood, G. M., & DiClemente, R. J. (1992). Cultural, gender, and psychosocial influences on HIV-related behavior of African-American female adolescents: Implications for the development of tailored prevention programs. *Ethnicity & Disease, 2*, 381–388.

Winkelstein, W., Samuel, M., Padian, N. S. (1987). The San Francisco Men's Health Study III: Reduction in human immunodeficiency virus transmission among homosexual/bisexual men, 1982-1986. *American Journal of Public Health, 77*, 685–689.

Working Group. (1994). *HIV preventive vaccines: Social, ethical, and political considerations for domestic efficacy trial.* Washington DC: Office of AIDS Research, National Institutes of Health.

Wright–DeAgüero, L. K., Gorsky, R. D., & Seeman, G. M. (1996). Cost of outreach for HIV prevention among drug users and youth at risk. *Drugs & Society, 9*, 185–197.

Yalom, I. D. (1985). *The theory and practice of group psychotherapy* (3rd ed.). New York: Basic Books.

Young, M., Core–Gebhart, P., & Marx, D. (1992). Abstinence-oriented sexuality education: Initial field tests of the Living Smart curriculum. *Family Planning Perspectives, 10*, 4–8.

Zenilman, J. M., Hook, E. W., & Shepherd, M. (1994). Alcohol and other substance use in STD clinic patients: Relationships with STDs and prevalent HIV infection. *Sexually Transmitted Diseases, 21*, 220–225.

Zuckerman, M. (1971). Dimensions of sensation seeking. *Journal of Consulting and Clinical Psychology, 36*, 45–52.

Zuckerman, M. (1994). *Biological expressions and biosocial bases of sensation seeking.* New York: Cambridge Press.

Author Index

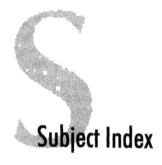

Subject Index